WHAT A LIFE CAN BE:
One Therapist's Take On Schizo-Affective Disorder
Based On A True Story
by
Carolyn Dobbins, PhD

Library and Archives Canada Cataloguing in Publication

Dobbins, Carolyn, 1960-
    What a life can be : one therapist's take on schizo-
affective
disorder : based on a true story / by Carolyn Dobbins.

ISBN 978-0-9866522-2-6

    1. Schizoaffective disorders--Patients--Biography.
2. Psychotherapist and patient. I. Title.

RC553.S34D62 2011   362.196'85810092   C2011-906422-7

First Published in 2011 by Bridgeross Communications,
Dundas, Ontario, Canada

For my
Mom and Dad...

Who have been there...
Who have taught me...
Who have applauded for me...

I thank you today.
I love you forever.

Disclaimer

This is a memoir rather than an autobiography. A memoir can be subjective, can leave things out and doesn't have to present every fact as does an autobiography. My memoir is *my* truth and is not necessarily *the* truth. Somewhere I read that many people witnessed an event, and there were as many versions as there were people.

Also, I have used some real names with people's permission. In other instances, the names are fictitious. I stayed away from naming agencies, mainly just to keep things simple. It also seemed that, in naming some, there would be people identified whom I thought were problematic. I wish no one ill will.

And so, feel free to agree or disagree with anything I say. E-mail me and let me know how you feel, because maybe then I can incorporate some kind of helpful response in a sequel. And remember, we all have our own *genius*. I hope you have found or find *yours*.

And, while I had much help in the editing, any errors or omissions are my responsibility.

carolyndobbins44@yahoo.com

Table of Contents

PROLOGUE

If I had any guts, I'd tell you about my life. In fact, one morning, I woke up and said to myself, "I'm going to write about *me*." Then, I thought, no, I'm rather uneventful. I hung with that thought all day long and decided, hey, maybe there's more to me than the eye can see.

***

Knoxville, Tennessee, where I live for now and maybe for a long time, suits me. No matter where I've lived, I've almost always been simple, broke and single. I am love, so I think. That makes me sound like a recycled hippie, which I am *not*. If anything, I'm one of those nerd intellects with a shy smile who didn't go on a date until age 16. I was *busy*.

Good or bad, I've played it safe almost all of my life. And popular or not, I'm a psychotherapist. I sit, listen a lot and say a few things in an obvious effort to help. My clients take risks for me, it seems. Especially one client. Her name is Jane. She soared past me in her gutsy, forgiving love of life on terms I'd never thought of. She grabbed hold of me emotionally and even met up with me spiritually, just her ideas of something bigger than "self" if only a "higher self".

She took the time to communicate with my commonplace mind. Who's the client here? She touched me for her sake, and that makes her the client. Maybe my boring way of living, though, gave her a place to come in for a landing and meet up with normalcy.

After a while, I realized that maybe I should write about *her* life and what it was like for me to be her therapist.

Interestingly, in our first session, Jane told me that she wanted to tell someone about her life, to help herself heal.

I saw in her life a wondrous and forgiving intensity that reflected love, hope and courage. She showed me pain and acceptance. I appreciate her travels unbelievably. I grew to admire her lot in life, naïve and innocent at times, and how she played her cards. I still do and always will appreciate her audacity. I don't know where she is; she stopped coming to her sessions. She said good-bye to me, but it seemed that *I* was not ready. She, herself, stopped needing psychotherapy while I was still trying to catch my breath.

The only thread that connects me to her is her writing. She poured out her heart, mind and soul to me on paper. She said that she wasn't able to look me in the eye and tell me her life. She said that people, even therapists, can get in the way of living. That really hit me hard; we think we know our purpose. I graduated from one of the best doctoral programs in the country and yet...

Recently, I was standing in my office and looking out the window. I slammed her chart, heavy with its burden on my desk. Bang! I was so angry. What was I supposed to do? I didn't know. Then through my anger came the tears and countless red lights where I've sat, idling, just still and in pain. I turned to her chart and reread my notes and her shared writings.

This is what it was *for me.*

CHAPTER ONE MEET JANE

When I was a teenager, I read all kinds of stories...and it helped me hang on...and gave me hope.

July 20, 2009

"Jane?" There is only one person in the waiting room, so it must be her. I extend my hand and notice that her grip is stronger than I expect. She's thin and small-boned but holds my hand tightly. I say hello, and she smiles. I wonder if she has expectations of me, as she follows me back to my office. I wonder if *I* have expectations of *her*.

So do you have a name?

"Oh, yes." I look at the floor and brush off a self-conscious laugh. "Carolyn. You can call me Carolyn. Or Dr. Dobbins." There is a silence. I sit and venture a glance at her face. She must be 45-50 years old, I wager. Yet she seems younger for some reason.

Who waters your plants?

"I think they're artificial."

Well, then, hopefully, no one waters them. Why are they artificial?

"They're made out of plastic."

That's not what I meant. I meant, why don't you have real plants in here?

"I really don't know."

I believe you. I, myself, think it might be an issue of nervousness.

"Oh?"

Yes.

"Nervousness?"

Yes. You'd make your clients nervous.

"How's that?"

You'd forget to water them. And then they'd droop. And then your clients would wonder if you're capable of keeping things alive, of helping people come alive and get healthy.

"Why do you think I'd forget to water them?"

You just don't seem like the plant-watering type.

"How do you figure that?"

Because you have artificial plants.

How did we get in this merry-go-round of an exchange? Feeling like an exposed idiot, I grasp at where to go from here. I am saved by Jane.

However, I, for one, think that plants and people differ. You seem like a people-person. Maybe you care more about people than you do plants.

"How do you figure that?"

Easy. You're not a botanist.

How do I ward off the next loop? Should I even be trying to? I sit and wait. I sneak a quick glance at my clock and then look back into Jane's eyes. She smiles and kicks the heel of her left tennis shoe into the rug.

"So where do we go from here?"

A botanical garden?

I smile. Jane sighs, and I sense the pain in her voice. She keeps it tucked away for only the astute. I tell her that I'd like to be there for her. Good, she says.

Well, seriously, I've led an interesting life, Dr. Dobbins. It hasn't been easy. I feel that there are a lot of loose threads and loose connections, lessons and claims to fame that I want to sort out and sift through. So I guess I just want to tell someone, just one person, my story. I'm hoping it will help me, you know, empower me. And yet, what I'd really like to do in that process is help someone else.

When I was a teenager, I read a lot of life stories of people who had endured all kinds of pain, and it helped me hang on. They gave me hope. They let me in -- just accounts of ordinary people or famous people, it didn't matter. I read a lot. My reading, though, has never been for pleasure. It has been to get information, to feel soothed and to have friends, to somehow relate.

Being a teenager is so hard, and for me, it seemed three times as hard. I think of the ones who are lost in our world, the ones who need help but don't know who to turn to. I just wish I could tell each and every one of them to hang in there, look for kindness and realize that pain doesn't have to last. You know, things can get better.

So I'd like to write a book or a story that might help someone along. It's about letting people who are unusual and off the beaten path believe that they have a place in this world. Dr. Dobbins, I've had my own doubts about myself. I have sometimes feared that I take up space that should not be mine. I'm not talking about being a pig. I am talking about the air we breathe.

Does she feel so unwanted?

Well, I want to write my story, and you tell me if it's worth reading. You tell me if I make sense. You pull it all together. I'll share my life with you, and you can bring it home. I don't want to be known. You can write a story based on truth, my truth. But leave me out of it.

So she has expectations of me. Does everyone want to write a book?

"Jane, maybe you just need to do what is helpful to you. In the here and now. The issue of a book, maybe that kind of decision-making can come later. You might change

10

your mind. You might want to write it all out and pull it all together yourself."

Yeah, maybe. I guess.

"You have come to me as a client. Psychotherapy often involves change. Your writing can be a vehicle, and you can give me anything you wish for me to read. In the process of meeting, though, we'll establish a relationship, a partnership. Through that, you might change."

You might change, too.

"Well, true. I'd be lying or in denial if I thought therapists were static in their work with people."

Jane leans back in her chair and takes a deep breath. She tells me that she wants to feel safe. She wants to trust me. She knows the ins and outs of therapy. She has been to therapists before. She tells me that a lot of therapists don't even have plants in their offices. I ask her what she means by that, why is that important. She says that if artificial plants have a place, maybe she does, too. She says that artificial plants make her feel more real. She calls it a "downward comparison."

"You have an interesting take on things."

Yeah, well, I can shut it off, too. When it comes to survival, you kind of learn what works and what doesn't. Maybe that's what I'm doing in the here and now. I've learned a whole lot about what works from being dragged through a whole lot of what doesn't. I've grown a whole lot in managing my life, in managing myself. I know what to say and what not to say. I know how to stay on track, you know, a process that works for me. I'm just saying that therapy should be a place where I find a freedom and a safety, a place where a person does not have to color within the lines quite so much.

"Look, Jane, this is your time. This is meant to be a

11

place where you can be whomever and whatever you wish. I'm not going to judge you. I'm sure you know of boundaries..."

They make the world go round, when people adhere to them.

Jane smiles. It sounds as if she's had a really rough go of things. I look at her as she looks out the window. She seems young at heart, and she seems to carry, literally, the weight of the world. How can I know her pain? Maybe I can't, but I can listen.

Dr. Dobbins. Hello?

I jump a bit, as Jane breaks into my reverie.

"I'm sorry. I was thinking."

Jane laughs.

A lot of people don't, you know. A lot of people don't think at all.

Jane places her elbows on her knees and then places her chin in the palms of her hands. She smiles.

What I was going to say is that I'd like to see you. I'd like to be your client, if that's okay.

"When did you decide that?"

I'm curious about this and may never return to a time when I can ask. Some things only come around once.

"When I saw your sincerity in our exchange about your plants. You didn't even try to defend yourself or criticize me. You just kind of went with it, the loop. Real or imagined, I think you could be there for someone.

"Real or imagined?"

Yeah. I think you might care.

"And maybe I do."

There is a pause. I am starting to understand things a bit.

So if I come in here, and I tell you my story, I want to feel proud, not less than. I wouldn't let you reduce me to some smaller size. I've been through that. Actually, it's something that can happen any time, if you're not careful. I think that you'll be decent to me, though. That's why. So will you work with me?

I nod. Jane says thanks. We discuss payment and times to meet. Jane wants to schedule week by week. I say okay. I ask her if she is working anywhere. She tells me that she's a tech at a treatment center. I ask her how it's going. She tells me it's a huge challenge. How so? I ask. Just trying to carve out an existence, she says quietly. She begins to cry. I hand her a paper towel. She is laughing a bit and crying, all rolled up in one.

Dr. Dobbins, I am not hell bent on regrets.

She wipes away her tears.

But my life is just way too much to live at times. And yet, it's also not enough. Always looking back at having made it, or not made it, never knowing what I'm going to have to go through in my future. All I have is now, and it's painful.

She tosses a wad of paper towel in the waste basket.

I don't know where to begin, but I've said enough for today. I'd like to go.

She gets up to leave and tells me to please charge her for reading anything she writes. I tell her whatever she writes is included in payment for her sessions. She tries to argue, and I walk to my door. I turn the door knob, and she walks into the hallway. So I'll see you next week, I say.

The rest of my day goes quickly. Between clients, my mind goes back to Jane. I'm not sure what to think of her yet, but I feel a stronger-than-usual desire to help her. Maybe I feel a bit of a kinship with her, although in some ways I think we're opposites. Things are so safe in my journey through life. There's such order and predictability. Or so it seems.

I drive home cautiously, wanting to be sure I don't get one of those camera-intersection traffic tickets. I pull in my driveway, ready for the best part of my day. I kick my shoes off, rip my clothes off, and jump into shorts and a T-shirt, all in one motion. Lady!

Lady usually greets me at the door. Not today. Hey! Sleeping on the job? Let's go! She stretches, waiting for me to say the word: "Truck?" She dances a jig of total joy. We hop in the truck and drive a few miles to a parking lot next to a bike trail. I hop out and grab my roller blades. Lady jumps through the window to the back of the truck and waits, looking on in anticipation and wagging her tail with complete glee.

Lady is sixteen years old but fast. She stops every now and then to mark her territory. I think she learned that from Bo, because I don't think many female dogs innately stop every ten yards to pee. I miss Bo. He was my problem child, a biter. He thrived on power and control but could be so sweet at the same time. Everyone thought that I should put him to sleep for biting, but I never did. Instead, I protected him from people. I didn't put him in a position to bite someone. I knew it had to be that way. And we had a wonderful life up until he got sick at age twelve or thirteen. He had arthritis and got to where he'd bite if I picked him up the wrong way. He bit me a few times throughout his life – either when he hurt physically, or when he thought I was trying to take his food from him. Then he got sick and soon after he died.

Even Lady, whom he pushed around a bit, grieved when he died. For months she sat in his favorite spots. She moped around and seemed genuinely sad. Only time put a dent in the pain. After that it was just Lady and me. We moved on. I tell Lady all the time that dog spelled backward is g-o-d. Are you my higher power, Lady? She buries her nose in the pillows. Grrr, I say, laughing. Why can't people be more like dogs?

Lady is all about food. I think she'd eat herself to death if she were provided an unlimited supply of hamburgers. She has even lunged at me and tried to grab my food. (She has done so successfully quite often.) She and I have an understanding at this point. Everything that makes her so important to me is based on an understanding – an understanding that I would throw myself in front of a car if it meant saving her life. I think I love her as much or more than anyone. She is just that important. She is just that good to me.

I see the selfish side in many people. I am one who can be taken for granted or taken advantage of by a lot of people. It's probably partly my own defect – that I pick the wrong people to be around. One thing I like about being a therapist is that I often am exposed to clients' vulnerable sides. I constantly pull for the good in them. My clients are often beaten down by life, even in extreme anger or deviance, and are just looking for someone who believes in them.

I'm a bit guarded in my personal life, but I'm always a believer. I try to learn and am always open to meeting up with a truly great person. I need to be cautious when I meet people; not everyone is good, and not everyone has my best interests at heart. And not all clients are easy.

The greatness of psychotherapy is that there are ethics, guidelines and boundaries that can bring out the best in people. I once had an adviser who told me that if he weren't married, he'd chase me all over the world just to have me. And I finally said to him, "Listen to yourself – if you had to chase me all over the world, what does that tell you?" He was speechless.

There is no room for this kind of sloppiness in dealing with our professional peers and colleagues. The framework of psychotherapy creates a safe playing field for the therapist, the therapist's peers, and the client, or at least it should. I do know this: I want to do right by my clients. And I want to be professional.

CHAPTER TWO WHERE TO BEGIN

I've been busy most of my life.

July 23, 2009

I walk in my office and reach for the light on my desk. I wonder what I've got going on for the day. I see Jane's name on my schedule. Am I going to be able to help her? What's going to unfold? I wonder these things and then am caught up with client after client. My confidence breaks free of doubt and carries me completely.

"Jane?" She makes eye contact and smiles. She follows me to my office as I ask how she's doing. Making it, she says. It's kind of a crap shoot, she says. How so, I ask, as I close my door, and we are alone. We are together, but we are alone, and it lasts for only fifty minutes.

I'm just not certain about a lot of things, like what I'm going to feel like when I go to bed, if I'll even sleep any, and what things will be like when I wake up. I'm not sure. And my waking hours, I'm lost in trying to figure out what kind of a day there might be for me. I know I can't move backward to a time when things were more secured. I have to go forward. What's it all worth? Do I even want to make a go of it?

"And you wouldn't, because? Things aren't secured?" I wonder what she means by that.

I'm tired. Tired of starting over. It gets old. Dr. Dobbins, I'm a really decent person, and I understand that a lot of decent people have lives paved with hell. The thing with me is that I don't even know how to explain my life. I see little meaning or purpose in it. It'd be great if something good could become of it, but the effort I make, the trauma I experience, what's the point? I guess I'm just tired.

"Jane, you're talking about reasons. Maybe you just don't see the reason right now – the reason you're here on this earth. Maybe there's a true-to-life reason you might come up with. Why not hang in there? Something worthwhile might be around the corner."

Well, then, I'm going to go ahead with my idea. I'm going to tell you about my life. It's the only thing I can hang onto. And I've never told anyone my story. It has always hurt too much to even breathe my past. I've always tried to outrun it, but that doesn't work anymore, Dr. Dobbins.

A tear runs down Jane's cheek. I want to reach toward her pain and say it's okay, but what if that doesn't help? How do we know when we're helping someone and when we aren't? I sit quietly and look at the mindless artificial plants. At least they belong in my office. And for this fifty minutes, Jane belongs with me. I owe her my best.

"Okay, so your story, yes?" I lean forward, hoping this might be another beginning for us. Yet Jane just sits and says nothing. Our silence is not a power struggle. She seems truly to be at a loss for an entrance into a meaningful relationship. I sit and wait. It feels like an hour that goes by. Then she shifts her weight sideways, looks down at her hands and says something, in a whisper.

Dr. Dobbins, I've never even painted my toe nails – started to one time when I was twelve or so. And I got distracted. I'm forever distracted. You know, a tomboy, an athlete, trying to go to school, my illness. I've been busy most of my life.

I listen with full intent to understand her. This is her process.

Well, I can start by saying that my life started out pretty well. I'm not going to take up time dissecting my childhood, because it was good. I knew I was loved. My parents provided my sister and me a lot of opportunity and gave us a lot of freedom. Denver, Colorado was an awesome place to grow up in the 60s. I was an adventuresome, smart, talented kid. I wanted to do the right things. Life was simple and straightforward. My parents instilled in me discipline, self-reliance, patience, the importance of education. They taught me that most things of value, you have to work for. Admittedly, though, I was a bit difficult, little things, like ignoring people I didn't like.

"Like who?"

People who tried to control me. Sometimes people who told me to do something I thought was wrong. Let's not go into it. I just think some people live wrong.

Jane takes a deep breath and exhales as if to take a timeout. I wait.

But some people really suffer. My parents were both health professionals (my dad a pediatrician and my mom a nurse), retired now, and I always wondered why some kids had it so tough when it comes to illness, poverty, broken homes. I mean, my childhood was great. School was great, although I got in trouble at times. I was involved in sports and music, had slumber parties, had pets...and looking back, I never would have made it as an adult without the stability and love my parents provided. I don't know what would have happened to me, but I wouldn't have made it.

Well, maybe if someone – anyone – had been there for me, I'd have made it. Yes, I think so. You don't have to have all of what I had to make it in life, but I was lucky. I do believe that just one person can make a difference. My parents, though, have helped me a lot. I think that I've been a tremendous burden.

I have an illness that has been tough to carry. It has saddened and worried my parents, and to escape it, they took trips, they had good lives. It was still rough on them, as they *cared immensely. My sister was never seriously exposed to it, and I made an effort not to put her in a position of having to help me. I remember one time banging my head against the wall and waking her up. After that, I tried to be as quiet and as invisible as possible.*

"Can you tell me more about what you think would have happened without help?"

I think I would have died. Not sure how, maybe exposure, to what I don't know. My parents always had a roof over our heads. They always extended that to me. Otherwise, I don't know. I guess I would have been homeless, which I've actually been at one time. Maybe someone would have helped me, maybe someone who works in a decent group home or shelter, maybe a foster family, maybe a therapist...or maybe I would have been raped and murdered.

Sometimes I think it would have been better if I had died in my teens. That makes me cringe. I dragged a lot of people through hardship, not of my doing. I couldn't help it. It has been hell for me, over and over. Where it's all leading to, maybe it'll seem worth it someday. Today, it's not worth it.

Jane seems troubled in her thoughts. I ask her if there were ever a time in her adulthood when things were good. She nods her head yes. Then maybe things can be good again, I say. Maybe, she says. I doubt it, she adds. This troubles me this time, because I don't know how to tell her about hope. It can be good again, I say with emphasis. It can be. She seems to ignore me and keeps talking. I stop talking.

Things didn't get really difficult for me until I was sixteen or seventeen years old or so. I was a top athlete, nationally-ranked quite high as a junior, in my teens – in several sports actually, the sky was the limit – lacrosse, field hockey, both Alpine and Nordic skiing. Mainly Alpine skiing and then Nordic when I was injured. I was very, very good and had so much potential. Plus cycling, and I grew up on a trampoline, where there was never any holding back. Doing flips from the roof...my mother cursed my pediatrician who said to get me interested in sports.

Honestly? I was heading for the Olympics, in 1980 and/or 1984 in skiing; I competed all over the world...and then it was as if a switch were thrown. Within months, I found myself in Boston, peddling on a stationary bicycle with a catheter in my arm. As I said, Dr. Dobbins, when I was 16, I was on a track heading for the 1980 Olympic Games in Lake Placid. I'm not just saying that.

The scientists at Massachusetts General Hospital told me that they thought I had a metabolic disorder. My morning resting pulse was 30 beats per minute, which is very low. I was producing an amount of lactic acid that was making me ill. Yet they really had no solutions. They told me that I tolerated lactic acid like they'd never seen.

My legs were heavy, like lead. My balance was off. I was dizzy. I was slow. I didn't know what was what. I'd jump on the trampoline and complain that the springs were shot. I'd play tennis and say that the racket needed new strings. I'd cross-country ski and complain about the wax being wrong. Then, I realized that it was me.

I didn't know where to turn. I disappeared from competition. I could not shake what had happened to me. I looked in the mirror one day, touched the glass with my fingers and begged myself to come back. I was gone. I was never the same after that. Never.

Friends told me that that's what it's like to become a woman. Other people told me that I was burned out. At age 17? No way. I was over a thousand miles away from my parents. I tried to go to college. I remember that first semester as if it were yesterday. My existence being peeled away from me, layer by layer, and I could do nothing about it. I couldn't explain to anyone what was happening.

"So a metabolic disorder?"

That's what they said at MGH. Only they wanted to keep me on a metabolic research ward to see what they might find. It really scared me, so I left. I stayed with friends, here and there, until it was time to start college in Vermont. I finished high school early, and I kept thinking back to age 14, 15, 16...and hoped that I would pull out of the agony and return to the way I had been. My parents were supportive over the phone. I had been so independent and self-reliant, traveling all over the world. No one ever thought that I would be thrown by much of anything. I was considered smooth and steady, very capable and a lot of common sense.

So I started college. Ever see an injured animal, how it retreats and hides, knowing it can't protect itself? That was me. I asked for a single room. I hardly ever ventured out to class. I was on academic probation at the end of the semester. And my IQ is pretty much as high as an IQ can be.

I threw away everything I had except for what I was wearing and a backpack that I stuffed with sweat clothes. I walked off the campus and stopped at the first sign that said 'hiring'. I dropped my backpack with a thud, felt like 150 pounds.

"Then what?"

Within minutes, I was working at a motel. I cleaned rooms and bused tables. I ate the leftover food from people's plates. I slept in the basement. I remember how hard and cold the cement floor felt every morning when my feet hit the floor. I told my parents that I was on the talent squad and was training with the US Ski Team, which had been true for the two years before.

22

Again, I kept hoping that I would pull out of this metabolic mess of a life.

I felt caged in, unable to compete alongside peers that I outdid so easily in the years before, unable to meet the demands of college. I didn't know what to do. I kept working at the motel, horrified with the idea that I would change people's beds forever. Yet I accepted that that was my life. I hid from anyone who tried to help me. People who knew me knew that there was something terribly wrong with me. I was afraid of people and help, and I'm not sure why. Not wanting to know how bad it might be?

I noticed that I couldn't even think normally. I ran myself into the ground, trying to snap out of it. I tried not exercising for weeks to see if that would help. I tried eating, not eating, sleeping, not sleeping – whatever I was fighting had very much to do with sleeping and eating.

After several months at the motel, I got this idea that my insides were rotting out, that I was dying. I felt physically horrible. The problem was that I couldn't figure out how to get to my parents who were over a thousand miles away. Should I hitchhike and just show up? They didn't have Map-Quest back then. I called my dad and asked him to get me a flight, something that I easily did for myself when I was in high school.

I remember the look on my dad's face when he picked me up at the airport. He literally turned white when he saw me. That was around 30 years ago. My life that had been amazing was gone. It was gone forever. I cried endlessly, as if every day I died. In some huge and incomprehensible way, I really had died. Sports had been like a best friend to me and then was gone. Forever. I never came close to having a full, highly successful sports career that was evolving with ease.

"So life as you knew it..."

Well, that was where my difficulty truly began. When I

23

returned to my parents, I was a fish out of water. I existed in Knoxville, Tennessee where my parents had moved to when I was fifteen years old. I knew no one. I was lost whenever I went outside. I was lost whenever I stayed inside. Dr. Dobbins, I was just plain lost.

Jane pauses. She tells me that she is at a stopping place. She thanks me for letting her rattle on. You aren't rattling on, I say. Feels like it, she says. She stands up and rides up on tiptoe. She holds herself in the poise for a moment and then eases herself down, flatfooted once again.

Dr. Dobbins, I'm going to start writing. You know what's hard? When I was living it, I didn't know that things were going to get worse and worse. I mean, I was just a 'kid' when all of this started. And writing about my life, well, I know things are going to get worse and worse. For a long time, they did. I think it's going to be really hard to write my story.

"Let me know what I can do to help." I say that with an immense feeling of helplessness. I will, she says. She thanks me.

"What are you thanking me for? I haven't really done anything yet."

Dr. Dobbins, remember Winnie the Pooh? One time, Piglet came up to Pooh and whispered, Pooh! Then Piglet said he didn't need anything from him; he just wanted to be sure of him.

"That's hope, Jane. I think that's hope." Maybe there's hope for a connection.

Well, I guess I know that, and that's what I'm thanking you for. Some therapists sleep through their sessions with clients. It seems your clients matter.

I am aghast. Leaving me there, Jane tiptoes out, saying Hush, and I break into a slight laugh.

I am on my way home. I see that the stop light will

24

probably turn yellow on me, and I speed up. Got through that, I think, no camera intersection ticket for me today, nope. Hope not anyway. Sometimes I think that I love motion, to be moving, because treading water is tough. I even enjoy moving a chess piece on a board. I love to play bridge, being able to remember what cards have been played. Finesse is a phenomenal thing.

With Jane, it really is going to be tough, though. I need to be still from moment to moment. This is her deal, her moves, her very life. I have hope for her courage, I'm thinking, as I pull around a corner and accelerate. I just want her to have some support, some relief -- in whatever way that is supposed to happen. I hurry a bit and look at my watch. It's not that late, and I decide to swing by my parents' house. They are old now, and I can close my eyes and almost touch their young adult faces, at a time when I was just a child.

I start to cry. I pull over and into a parking lot that houses a vacant building. This is where a toy store was once filled with excitement and wonder. This really sucks, aging sucks. Change sucks. Time sucks. Everything sucks.

I join my parents in their den. They ask me how things are going. They are going, I say with a smile. I tell them a little about Jane and how atypical her plan is, to put her life on paper as a form of therapy. People do that, I tell my parents. It's just that her reason for doing so is because she doesn't want a therapist to get in the way. So why is she seeing you? my mom asks. To have someone there, I say. Just to have someone there. You never know what might help, Mom. I just want to help, I say. Yeah, we know, my parents say in unison. Hmm, well, they know me, which is comforting.

Then something in me floats to the surface. Feeling compelled to know, and out of the blue, I ask my parents if I have done okay. As a daughter. Underneath, I am thinking about Jane, her comment about dragging people through things. Kids and parents drag each other through things, in varying ways. My parents look at me as if I've caught them off guard. Oh my, of course you have, they respond. You've done better than okay. So have you, I say.

I drive home thoughtfully, run outside and back in with Lady quickly. I vaguely remember falling asleep, thinking over Jane's comments about food and sleep. Then I go somewhere else in my mind and let go. Time stands still. It is morning.

July 24, 2009

I'm running a bit behind schedule with a heavy load today. I get the feeling that Jane's effort to look at herself and her life sets me up to take a closer look at myself. I've chosen boring over adventure, and yet I respect people so much who take a stand and put themselves out there. I've always felt like the most enthusiastic bystander. I don't know why I've been the observer and not the player. Yet I've always felt busy and filled with life on life's terms.

I've been there for my most important friends who've been through those most important experiences. I've witnessed births and deaths and weddings. I've followed people all over the country just being there for them – for sporting events, when they win scholarships, when they graduate from schools and colleges, when they need a friend, when they retire.

I think I'm prepared to walk with Jane through her account of her life. Though I hardly know her, I sense that

26

her story carries importance. I wonder what has transpired over the past thirty or more years.

Yes, Jane seems important, extremely rich in a philosophical way. I can't quite put my finger on it. She has started to portray a sort of ruggedness and quiet power emanating from her, perhaps. It's as if she knows a lot of things I don't know, but she comes across as humble. She seems controlling, but I think this might be her need to be in control. She's not trying to control me, she's just "hell bent" on making sure that she stays in control of herself. There's a difference.

I sit in my office, twirling a pen in my hand and tapping on my desk calendar. Look at my pens! Lexapro, Abilify, Geodon, Effexor, a drug holiday just sitting before me in an amazement. 2009, and whoompsh! Psychotropic drugs everywhere. Here's another: Celexa. And another: Paxil. Do these pens even write? I don't know! Drugs are everywhere these days. Prescriptions, street drugs, jacked up beverages, flavored beers, the list is endless.

Is this the paved road to immediate gratification? I am so simple and settled that I don't even have credit cards, and I don't know how to send a text message. Yet I am quite content with that. I listen to oldies rock and traditional country in my car, almost convinced that it's still the 60s.

Pens or no pens, I do exceedingly well with clients in that I try to build sincerity around them. Jane asks that I trust her to be seeing a physician and taking care of herself medically, that she doesn't want to go into all of that right now. Somehow, I do trust her. Sometimes I think it's best to let things unfold a bit or evolve, without forcing issues.

Truly caring about clients, human beings, carries me

far into a land where love conquers all. Being unconditionally loving builds a bridge for them to walk across into their new lives. They get a glimpse of who they want to be, and then go for it. Confidence follows when what a person wants deep inside shines through and true. I don't want to squash these all-important developments. Sometimes it's best to step back a bit. Sometimes it helps when we watch someone on a high wire with no net, but I'm not sure how or why it helps. For me, it always matters when they make it to safety. The relief can be stupendous.

I fully recognize that this doesn't sound like intricate, research-based psychological theory. I'm comfortable knowing all of those things. I just think that we humans are all searching for something quick and magical. We confuse ourselves, yet it really boils down to wanting to be loved. I truly believe that even the most hardened people, in their calloused way, are still just looking for love.

CHAPTER THREE THREE YEARS OF HELL

Sorry, Mom and Dad, but I can't take it any more.

Several days go by quickly. I'm concerned about my parents. They are forgetful, slow. I try to swing by for a visit at least every other day. They like to watch movies, and it's something we can do together. Now and then, we see a great one, typically based on a true story. A great story unfolds when someone puts his or her heart on the line to help a child. Or a prisoner. Or a very tired mother with too many mouths to feed. A great story happens when someone helps another person just because help is needed. Sincerity touches my heart.

For a true story to be meaningful, it must somehow display how love works, how fear can be overcome. That brings tears to my eyes. And when the story is based on truth, it's so remarkable to see faith-building operations, hope and honor for one another. Love matters in people's lives. It's our job to allow this, to promote this. To me, this is our *job*, really, no matter our employment situations.

***

Jane is a no-show. My receptionist, however, hands me a large envelope with a stack of pages inside. Jane has scribbled me a note that rests on top.

Sorry to miss my session. Here's my payment. Will you read this? I scheduled with your receptionist, and I'll see you next week.

I am hit with sadness and frustration. Why can't she talk with me? Have past therapists really been that negligent? We are supposed to be something other than a burden. This woman can barely bring herself to recite her experiences. What was it she said – that she would have given up? She would have retired to a rocking chair by a window at age twenty? She almost ditched us, and maybe she has a point. Maybe we've unknowingly hurt her, and she's grown cautious and wise. And so she won't let us hurt her, yet she still needs us?

I drive straight home after a whirlwind of a day. I like my clients. I admire their courage. With Jane, I have perhaps overstepped a boundary, being too interested in her. It's not even that I like her, but she really seems to need a break. I try stepping one foot into all of my clients' realities. Jane seems guarded, resistant in a way. She is not trying to manipulate me with her writing, but she is genuinely afraid of me. I wonder if someday I might meet her in the middle. I hope so.

I take Lady roller-blading. She runs beside me, keeping good pace for a couple of miles, surely thinking about the hamburger she's going to devour on the way home. She loves me, and she loves drive-thru restaurants. When the voice wants to take our order, she's a new dog, literally jumping up and down. It's that simple with her. I love everything about her.

No hamburger today, *can't* have one every day, sweetie, I tell her, your blood work, Lady, it's great, and we're going to keep it that way...She ignores me. We rush home and up the stairs. She beats me to the pillow on the bed. No fair, I shout. She does this jerking motion with her back legs, wanting to play. Calm down, I say. She hops off the bed and digs a nest in her blue and yellow Scooby-Doo comforter on the floor. I think it's like a victory tour to her. And I think she knows how cute she is.

30

I grab my overcrowded purse and sling it on the bed. There must be twenty dollars of change in here, I think. Six lipstick tubes, stale gum. Here we go: I slide the large brown envelope that encases Jane's writing across my legs. I try to stay in shape. My feet are soon to be 50 years old. Same goes for the rest of me. I laugh with myself. My cell phone rings. Not recognizing the number, I let it go and start to read.

Jane is writing in the present tense. I wonder why. I picture her in a room that has nothing familiar except for the furniture. It's not as if someone else has moved into her being. No, she makes it clear that she knows the girl she has lost. That perfectly-trained, athletic-driven adolescent is gone, and Jane knows that painful reality. She writes:

Am I nineteen years old? Twenty? How many months did I wander around? How many beds did I change? How many plates did I clear? I make my way down an unfamiliar hallway in a very unfamiliar house and city...and turn into the bathroom. I can't bring myself to look in the mirror. I have done that before, and it devastates me.

My hands are puffy. My muscles sag. I try to stand up straight and tall, holding onto the sink to catch my balance. I feel as if I am going to pass out. I drop to my knees and just rest there for a long moment. I need to go back to bed. I drink a glass of water and head to a room that is now mine, at the end of a dark hallway that approaches a desolate eternity.

I do this repeatedly, for days. The bathroom, the hallway, my room – it's all a bad dream. Some days, I try for the kitchen. I sit slumped at the table across from the refrigerator and talk with my mom. She may not know what it was like, traveling all over the world. Yet surely she knows my energy as a child and the times we visited when my schedule allowed. She seems worried and tells me that time might heal these aches and pains of mine. When my dad comes home each evening, he says very little. My parents fret.

I bet weeks and months go by, and nothing. No change. No answers. I find that I cannot take this existence any longer. I think it's been two or three years of having periods. So is this hormonal? I was slow to actually head into adolescence. I wish I could go back to age 15 or 16. Nothing helps. This is adulthood? Do other people feel this way? What keeps them going? I want to die.

I find a pad of paper and a pen. I creep downstairs and lie down on my stomach in the den. The carpet scratches my legs. It's annoying as I write a letter to my parents: Sorry, Mom and Dad, but I can't take it anymore. Three years of total hell is all I can do. I love you, Jane.

It seems both frightening and peaceful to figure out how to do it. Why stay alive if I feel like this? My mom walks in and asks what I'm doing. Nothing, I lie. I'm crying. Then I start bawling my eyes out. She hugs me. She takes the note and reads it. And then she starts to cry, too. My dad says that suicide is a permanent solution to a temporary problem. Things can change, he says, please be patient. Hmm.

My parents have an advantage when it comes to genetics. They know their parents' lives. They know their cousins and aunts and uncles. I never knew some of these relatives as completely crazy, just different. I found them interesting and enjoyed talking with them.

I guess enough time has gone by and enough action on my part that it sends my dad on a search for the right doctor who might help me. I am clueless, and my parents' conversation is quiet and serious. I'm glad that I can't hear what they're discussing, as I lie on my bed in my room. Yet I know.

My dad comes in and talks with me. A psychiatrist? I scream. You want me to see a shrink? I ask my dad. Get out, get out of my room! I exhaust myself in my own self-induced disaster. My dad's ready for me. He hands me a paper on biochemistry. I wad it up and throw it against the window. A housefly would have more impact. Calm down, my dad whispers. I sob.

Hours later, I wake up. My eyes are swollen. I crawl to the edge of my bed and reach out with my finger tips until they grasp the article. I straighten out the wrinkles and read. I get my first of a long series of explanations about neurotransmitters. I lie back against the headboard of one twin bed and after a time hear myself faintly snoring. I wake up in the middle of the evening, never knowing what time it is. I roll off the bed and crawl into the closet to counter some feeling of being totally overwhelmed. Nowhere is the only place I know to hide. From myself?

The next day is here. I do my best to study the article. It's actually a pharmacology bulletin on the chemistry of depression. Explained that way, as if depression can be chemical, it makes a bit of sense. I remember when I was barely 16 years old, I said that I could do anything I put my mind to. Where does that leave me if my mind is incapable of thinking, focusing and concentrating? Where does that leave me if my mind is utterly disarrayed, beyond the power of will?

I see my dad pull in the driveway. I wait for him to come through the door. I try not to bother him, as I hear him set his keys on the dresser in my parents' room. I know I need someone more than ever before. I am so afraid. I sit on my bed and drift off, waiting for my dad to come in my room and talk with me. He says hi, hang in there. Several more weeks go by.

My mom comes in my room. We talk for days, as I lie with my feet propped above my head against the wall. She tells me that

Dad wants to be absolutely certain about sending me to a psychiatrist. Meanwhile, I keep seeing an internist who runs tests after tests on me. I, myself, am still perplexed about lactic acid and my metabolic uncertainty. I don't understand any of it. I am always exhausted, wanting to care but not having the energy.

I find myself sleeping hours upon hours, and this has gone on for over three years. The internist sets me up for a sleep study. The lab technician tells me to stay awake all night so I'll be able to sleep in the lab the next day. I can't do that; I cry. My parents become my worst enemies as they pat me to help me keep my eyes open. I scream. I kick. This is killing me. They are relentless. I would rather be dead.

Then I look up at the clock in the kitchen. I touch my arms with my hands. The clock's hands, my hands, racing round and round...I feel a clarity for a moment. Then I feel my head spinning out of control, and I stop my mind with a screwy suddenness. This is too much, but I stop crying. I tell my parents that I won't be having any trouble staying awake until morning. I go downstairs and jump rope to The Rolling Stones until dawn. I don't sleep again for a week.

Abruptly, I come to the end of Jane's typing. I have an idea of what she was going through. I feel so incredibly sad for her. She was just a kid, no earthly idea what she might have been up against. Even in the 80's, biological psychiatry was in its infancy. If a person had a short bout with depression, his or her career was pretty much over. Jane's sports career was over, it seemed, but her life hadn't even begun. What kind of a chance did she have with depression, especially back then?

At least she had herself. What a great person to have in her corner. I silently ask her to hang on, because we all have an inner version of ourselves at every age. We mustn't

34

forget who we've been, especially if it helps us stay in the fight. Maybe if she could just remember herself as a child, or an undying curiosity over the final chapter in a book, one that *might* have a happy ending.

I am limited in my biochemistry know-how, and maybe it's a dead end for Jane to see a psychiatrist. What if it doesn't help? I don't see an easy way out of what destiny there is in her life. Jane tells me too much for me to hope for that. Her raw grit is going to write thirty or more years' worth of a life. I'm too tired to think, which is a blessing.

***

August 6, 2009

When Jane comes to see me, I feel ready. I ask her what happened with the sleep study and the lab tests. Did you ever see a psychiatrist? What about your metabolism? Slow down, she tells me. There was nothing straightforward, Jane says.

I tell myself, frankly, to shut up. Jane tries snapping a leaf off my plant. Dr. Dobbins, neither one of us is artificial, she says, facing the window with her legs hanging over the far side of her chair. We're both real. So...are we making progress, I ask. Well, I appreciate your enthusiasm, Dr. Dobbins, she whispers, but it wears on me. I am fighting for my life these days, and I need you.

I look at her, only to see her huge, sad blue eyes telling me more about her pain than words ever could. I am so sorry, I say. I'm trying to tell you something, will you just listen? she asks. It becomes quiet. She lets go of the plant. Five entire minutes go by, and Jane says thank you with an innocence I won't forget. I'm learning patience.

Dr. Dobbins, writing about my life is really difficult. It's often agonizing to be alone, and it's agonizing to talk about my

35

life. I'm starting to think that I can't do this. I can't write about my life. And with it being so depressing to me, who would ever want to read it, you know? I have lost a sense of purpose, because I really do want to heal. Yet I can't seem to take that step.

And the thing is, my life never really got much better once I had to quit sports. I think I mainly adjusted quite a bit. I learned to deal with it, and I wouldn't know how to even begin to explain myself and what I do that allows me to cope. My life has been my meager efforts to try to land a damaged plane, to go through the burn manually, every minute.

I guess I need to come in here and make sure that I keep moving. I need to keep growing for today and for a better tomorrow. And maybe talking with you will help me put my past on paper. I think I do want to do this. I tell myself that there's a light at the end of the tunnel. Seeing is believing, but sometimes you have to believe in order to see. Actually, I think we're supposed to let our own lights shine, but I'd like to know where mine went when I was a teenager.

I look at Jane and see her integrity, her tenacity. I say, What next from here? All right, so it's your move, she says. I squint my eyes as the sun starts coming through the window. I'm at a loss for words. Okay, Jane, I say, so push through the pain. What happened with the sleep study? She's reluctant but continues.

Nothing ever came of the sleep study. I never went to sleep in the lab. They even had me stay awake three days, and I still couldn't go to sleep in the lab, awake for a damn week. I found the only thing that could jolt me out of the insomnia was consuming just about everything in the refrigerator and cupboards. I ate boxes of cereal, drank maple syrup and wolfed down a gallon of ice cream. Then I crashed, exhausted and ill. The agony, carbohydrates and tryptophan, I guess, seemed to ground me.

Then they did a five-hour glucose tolerance test on me, and I couldn't eat for a day or something. I remember feeling shaky, and I stood up at one point and looked in a mirror. I could not even see myself, but I could see the mirror. The biochemist brushed that one off. Nothing came of anything except that they said my insulin overshoots, causing my blood sugar to drop low. So nothing was getting me even a back seat on the bus, not that day. I only knew that my problems had to do with sleep and food – either they were symptoms or part of treatment or both.

So several weeks went by, and I think that seeing a psychiatrist weighed heavily on my dad's mind. He wanted to find the best, someone who practiced biological psychiatry. So the next thing I knew, I was in a waiting room, thumbing through a magazine. I closed my eyes and saw myself. I was running in meadows and woods in my mind, up and down hiking trails...and to a deadening stop. Not even a damned reflection in a mirror!

Jane stops talking. Venturing further, I ask Jane if there is anything I can possibly do to make her life better today. Yeah, I went from having a metabolic disorder to sitting in a psychiatrist's waiting room, she says. Help me find my *home*. My God, I'm realizing, she just wants to belong.

Yet I didn't change just by walking through the door. It's just how you want to cut the cards. When I ate a lot of food, I had that feeling that doctors call depression. Coaches always wanted us to eat, eat, eat, so it's as if I ate my way into a long-standing depression, too much sleep, too much food, lethargic. And during those years, age 16 to 17, things about me were changing. I wouldn't really know how to explain it, but I'll tell you what I know about what happened to me. I'd say my problem is a complex, metabolic disaster. Call it whatever you want to call it, but the mechanism doesn't change.

37

Anyway, Dr. Dobbins, I sort of know what works for me. It has taken me 33 years to say that maybe I have arrived somewhere that seems fairly stable or quite knowledgeable about me in some ways. It's always been rough. But I know some things that are, honestly, of great value. And not just to me. I'm just not sure how to convey what I know.

So I have some kind of a genius on my hands, I think. Great. Admire her, respect her, love her. She needs you, Carolyn, I tell myself. Jane needs someone who can embrace an invitation to come into her heart. She won't judge you unless you judge her. Her door is open, and her troubles are *real*. Don't blow it, I tell myself. Be honest, open-minded and willing.

CHAPTER FOUR COLLEGE AGAIN

My parents don't have the answer. They didn't make me sick, and they can't make me well.

I imagine I'll hear from Jane soon. She seems pretty serious about her story. I am trying to figure out just how I can help with her idea about myths. Before she left last session, she said something about *having* an illness as opposed to *being* an illness. Are you a diabetic, or do you have diabetes? Are you a schizophrenic, or do you have the illness of schizophrenia?

She also mentioned stereotyping. That would involve the notion that all diabetics or schizophrenics have the same personality traits, the same something. At least, that's how she explained it. When a person has a mental disorder, it gets confusing. The symptoms of a mental disorder are often actual behaviors. And that nudges up next to personality. In fact, there is a class of mental disorders that are called personality disorders.

Jane's illness sounds like a "chemical imbalance". I read about a metabolic disorder called Phenylketonuria (PKU) in college, which was once considered a type of schizophrenia. In fact, in the case of PKU, there is a missing enzyme that prevents phenylalanine from converting to tyrosine. Interestingly, this is the metabolic pathway that allows dopamine to be made. And dopamine has a whole lot to do with mental illness.

Also, in the case of PKU, without the enzyme, there is a toxic product manufactured that can cause brain damage. So even though this is a gross simplification, it's worth thinking about. Reducing certain mental illnesses down to chemistry, in a way that promotes a reasonable level of control and understanding, might help people eradicate the myths. People with diabetes used to be housed in mental institutions. And people were probably afraid of diabetics back then, if only due to not knowing what was going on with them or what could be done to help them.

There is a new surge concerning psychotropic medications. This is a good thing, because it poses some answers, even if it's overdone these days. This is not how it was in the early 80s when Jane first saw a psychiatrist. There's still too much stigma, though, when it comes to the toughest mental illnesses. That's the unfair reality. It's complex, but it doesn't have to be that way. We need to move forward, address the confusions with great seriousness and replace the fears with *love* and *knowledge*.

I scribble on my desk pad. I wonder what the deal is with Jane. I'm sad, because she doesn't deserve whatever she's up against. It's late, and I'm tired.

***

August 14, 2009

It's been a while since I've heard from Jane. My keys rattle as I fumble for the one with the plastic coating. There are people in this world who work in a factory that makes these plastic covers for keys. I wonder what their lives involve. When I was a kid, I kept hoping that other kids had it good. For the most part, I had it good.

I walk down the hall and into my office. This is mine, this is me. I bought the rug, the furniture. Do I realize how lucky I am? I don't know. I cross the threshold and almost step on an envelope. My receptionist must have slid it under the door. I'm half-hoping it's from Jane. It is. I rip

40

through the seal the way I wish I could rip through her pain.

Dear Dr. Dobbins,

The only way I know to express what has happened to me when I was a very young adult is to go back and hold onto me. I must say that I had no clue what I was up against. Good thing.

My sports career landed me some medals and awards, but my career was cut way short. I was one of the best young, up-and-coming athletes in the nation and had such potential, and bang, game over, nowhere near a peak of any kind. However, my sports career did a lot for me that was invaluable. It taught me to hang on and push through and pull back. It taught me discipline, how to be a proud American (no matter the stigma that was developing) and how to use my intensity to my advantage. My sports career saved my life. It gave me a profound relationship with myself: never give up, never give in, be smart, stay focused. I'm a big believer in sports, in motion.

So there I was at age 19, maybe 20, flunked out of college, making beds in motel rooms, thinking I was dying – and in many ways I was – and then at my parents' place, in a big city and a house unknown to me, and I grabbed hold of something I thought would keep me alive: another chance at school. University of Tennessee was just ten miles down the road. I still was sleeping in my closet, anything to keep things simple and contained, but I wanted to go for it. I was afraid, so afraid that I would kill myself if I didn't have something to hang onto. Too much of me was gone for me to hang on. I wanted to still have a chance at an education. So I did. I tried. Meet Jane, at age 20 or so.

***

So what am I looking at? My sleep is as screwed up as ever. There's no normalcy, just confusion. And I can't figure out food to save my life. There's something in food that doesn't work for me. There's something in food that does work for me.

I decide I am going to try college again. I get the entrance forms. I fill them out and send them in. I'm accepted. I'm sure half the world is accepted, so no big deal. But most kids don't feel as utterly sick as I do. It's a very personal fight that no one seems to understand. Yet I fully know that others my age have already offed themselves, and I hurt terribly over this.

Meanwhile, I meet Dr. Jobson. He's the psychiatrist my dad worked hard to find. He's nice, and he takes my history. He wants to try lithium and an anti-depressant. Okay, I say. I'm dead tired. I wake up more tired than when I drop myself in a pile every afternoon. He's nice, though. Dr. Jobson is nice.

Weeks go by. Months go by, and the drugs aren't helping. Dr. Jobson says I can go to Boston if needed. Well, do you have a map? I ask him, in sheer desperation. I feel stuck rolling that boulder up that hill forever and all by myself. What a loser, seeing a psychiatrist. I turn in my rights. In Nazi Germany, I wouldn't have even made it to a concentration camp. Yes, they used to shoot people like me. I think there are situations when they still do. And that's not good.

It's when I walk in his office, a p-s-y-c-h-i-a-t-r-i-s-t'-s office, that I do change. I apply what I know of societal rules: I'm violent, I'm a basket case, there's no hope, lock me up and toss the key...how did I change from walking through the door? I don't know, but I, for one, don't think I actually did. It's a confusing issue. Meeting Dr. Jobson was embarrassing, disappointing, ridiculous and awful but no going back. That was the problem, I couldn't erase my chart or his notes. I even felt as if I had done something wrong. There went my innocence, over a shrink.

Do I have to lie down on the couch? I ask. No, he says. I guess I've lost a career in politics, huh? He smiles. What other limits or teen-age problems are suddenly assigned to me? It's all over for me, I think. I am 20 years old, but I feel 14, developmentally. What's happening?

It's Christmas, and my mom asks me if I want to make a fruit cake for Dr. Jobson. I say, Mom, he won't eat it. Why? she asks. Mom, don't you get it, I'm a mental patient now, and he's going to think I poisoned it or something. Where do you get that idea? she asks. From everywhere, I say, everywhere.

How am I going to register for school? Well, I won't know unless I get there. My parents are lost. Those books on kids written by psychologists don't seem to apply. Maybe as a way of coping, I find my mother throwing those books off the shelves and slam into the garbage. Seems they left out a few chapters which seemed to cause her undeniable distress. Yes, my parents are beside themselves. They think they are responsible. And they don't have the power they want. They didn't make me sick, and they can't make me well.

I am dying a little every day. I've got to do something. I grab hold of the university undergraduate catalog and start to cry, but no tears come. I lie on my bed. Then tears just start rolling and rolling down my cheeks. What is to become of me? I can't face an entire lifetime; I can't stand the gut-wrenching pain that long. This is physical pain.

I need to figure out how to register. My parents don't really know. Onward. My mom says maybe I've got a virus. Are you trying to be funny, Mom? I ask. No, she answers. In my own mind, though, I've been marked, a tattoo, an inked in number. I've seen a psychiatrist. My thoughts are simply always going, sometimes slowly, sometimes quickly, but always sideways, like treading water and never getting anywhere. I try to explain: Dr. Jobson, I am struggling, overwhelmed and confused all the time. Part of me lives for my appointments with him. His kindness is real and heartfelt. Mainly, I want an answer.

43

I ask my dad to drop me off at school. Let's go, he says, we'll give it a try. He looks worried. I say, five more minutes. He asks me how I plan on pulling this off if I can't even get up. I tell him I don't know, but it's not time yet. He waits in the car, motionless. We're quiet as he pulls into the circle in front of the administration building. Good luck, he says. I give him a hug. I guess, under the circumstances, even dads who are physicians are allowed to look lost, or especially to look lost. He let me go, to his credit.

The campus is huge. I'm just a particle in the grand scheme. There's a line of students that wraps around the entire building, twice. I get in line and feel like I'm going to pass out. I start to cry. Going to school seemed like a good idea at the time I thought about it. Yet this is for real. That problem happens to me a lot.

I get out of line and go inside. I duck into the ladies room and lock myself in a stall. I sit in there all day, trying to muster enough strength to get back in line. I pull my social security card out of my pocket. I have managed to hang onto it for eight years. I take a deep breath. I wipe my eyes and picture the line, knowing I need to get back at the tail end. I lunge out of the door. There is no line.

There is a lady standing at the entrance to a room with computers. She looks at my ID and directs me to someone who prints my schedule. I'm trying to figure out why I signed up for 1) English, 2) Nutrition, 3) Economics, 4) Psychology, and 5) Speech. Well, I have trouble with 1) language, 2) eating, 3) paying for things, 4) behaving, and 5) talking. Makes perfect sense. I make it through registration, relieved that no one asks me much of anything of importance. Just my name, and I can usually get that right. And my social security number, the card wadded up in my hand.

*I get a day off before I go to class. Phew, I need it.
Registration will always be stressful. So my dad drops me off and
picks me up in a fashion that becomes our usual pattern. I can
keep things straight, because my pick-up spot is right in front of
the Drop-Add door. Drop me off, pick me up. My mind is busy
and filled with disarray. It forms connections that make my
explanations sound crazy.*

*I'm looking for Economics 101. A girl stops and points
and jabbers. I am still lost, but I say thank you. Thank you for
caring. I find economics by sheer accident, but the guy has a
thick, foreign accent. I make my way to Drop-and-Add. All I
wanted was to learn to balance a check book if I ever get a job, I
tell the lady. She suggests Art History 101. Later when I walk out
of that lecture hall, I'm steaming. That's an easy A? All those
pictures projected up against the wall would give anyone a
headache. I end up sticking with just four classes. Maybe that's
enough.*

*I decide to eat a donut around noon. A bell sounds, time
for the next class, and I salivate. How funny! It reminds me I
need to scurry through the maze and make my way to Psychology
101. Salivate? Teach a pigeon to bowl? The only time I tried
bowling, I couldn't find the same size shoes, one left and one
right. One time, I tossed the bowling ball down the wrong alley.
How dumb am I, that I'd need a pigeon to teach me to bowl. And
some international athlete, jeez. So these realizations are stressful,
and this mental process happens all the time. I make connections
that most people don't comprehend.*

*In Nutrition 101, I sign up for an experiment about potato
chips. No kidding, I think they invent a spin-off of ruffled ones
that year. I not only test-taste the potato chips, I write a book
report on them and get an A. I turn in the same report for English
and get a B+. It was the same book report, how can that be?*

45

Which is it? Okay, I'll settle for an A-. Fair enough.

I don't know who is more puzzled by me: my parents, Dr. Jobson or me. I get all A's on my transcript for over a year. I decide I want to be a physician. My parents just look at me in exasperation and say, what? What? No one is amused or happy, that's for sure. And man, I was trying so hard, in my own way. My dad forgets to pick me up one day, and I tell him that he can work on remembering me. I'll work on getting into medical school. I even tape a reminder note on the steering wheel for him. He does not appreciate the help I try to provide him.

Among the A's, I wear sweat clothes and sneakers, no socks. I rarely take a bath, and I don't know why. Maybe too many other things to deal with. Yet somehow I adjust to myself. What I mean is that I learn to seem normal. I know I can't run or bike the way I once did, but I can tolerate the lactic acid. Yep, I get a gold medal for that. I want to finish college in the West. I dream of mountains, streams and hiking trails. I ditch the medication, which for two years, has given me nothing but a dry mouth and blurred vision.

CHAPTER FIVE 100 PRAYERS

My doctor told me that when I'm on, I knock the ball right out of the park.

I'm at home propped up against my bed with a huge pillow. I'm thinking that I know of a study in England where sleep deprivation has helped some people with depression. I vaguely remember hearing of that at a seminar I attended for continuing education units. Interesting how Jane snapped out of her hypersomnia when she was *made* to stay awake. Yet it was too much for her. She shifted into an existence where she hallucinated, the hands of the clock racing round and round. Then finally, to counter-balance the insomnia that went on for a week, she ate herself into a resting place, which was nothing of the sorts. It might have felt safer, more grounded, but it made her ill.

I rub my eyes and let my mind relax, which comes easily for me. I close my eyes and picture Jane's smile. I'd love to help her, but I know so little about her problem – if part of it is nutrition science, even if part of it isn't. She told me her internist decided that her trouble with food and sleep – her obsessions over never knowing what to eat and always having trouble with sleep – were all *symptoms* of an obsessive disorder. As though her ideas are invalid? He also said she had an attitude problem concerning her comment in response to his theory. She told him, rather matter-of factly, that he must have gotten through medical school on dumb luck. He wasn't happy, but that's Jane; she'll say what she thinks when she thinks it's the right thing to say.

Jane told me that she began doing her own reading. She came across an article where a handful of severely depressed patients didn't respond to medication but were helped by a diet loaded with tyrosine. Tyrosine is an amino acid that is found in protein and that is also converted from phenylalanine to dopamine. PKU, dopamine, mental illness, metabolic disorders – what's the connection? It was all very confusing to her.

I think that it was after these sessions where she seemed to be onto something that I started praying like crazy for her. Just in case it might help. Jane has the humility of *wanting* what she *gets*. But will she ever *get* what she *wants*?

She just wants to be good, that's all, just a good person. I laugh a little to myself about pigeons bowling and salivating over a donut, or a bell sounding. I get lost in what feels like a wandering prayer and fall asleep to the sound of the fan that I have propped against Lady's pillow. She likes the air on her face, and I like how it drowns out noises as I'm falling asleep.

***

It's morning, and I'm running late. I hop up and down on one foot and then the other, trying to slap on a pair of sandals. I drive safely but quickly, feeling focused and hurried by the clock below my dashboard. Wake up, I tell myself with enthusiasm; it's going to be whatever kind of a day there is in store! I park perfectly and race to the door right as Jane is pulling up. Good morning, she says. I wait a moment and open the door for her. She smiles. Come on back, I motion with my hand. Well, I'm reading what you're writing, I say. Yeah? she asks. It's quiet as I flip on the light.

I have more to come, Dr. Dobbins. I get depressed - in the feeling sense of the word, you know, an adjective. I write five minutes and then have to stop. I don't like grieving, but maybe I'm at least going somewhere! I've missed out on so much, Dr. Dobbins. Too much. And for what? I want to reach around and give the seventeen year old in me a huge hug. I had such guts. I was so clueless. I still am, but I just, I don't know, I find life to be a moment by moment thing.

"Can you tell me more about that?"

I live in the here and now. Everything I do is an effort to feel well, centered, tuned in...um, just hanging on and trying to reach some functional level of living. It's especially hard to do that when I'm trying to hold down a job. I've got to be 'on'. I've gotten better at that over the decades of living with myself. It's an ongoing test and chance to improve, every moment. I do amazingly well, though.

"Good for you, to your credit. I mean, my gosh, Jane."

Jane pauses. I sit patiently, then start to say, "You know, you really..." Jane interrupts.

I saw my doctor yesterday. I've known him for thirty years. So many of my efforts have been for me to have a life. Most people have a life and then go from there. I'm never ever there. I pass by Normal every now and then. Whoops, a moment of feeling well and thinking clearly. I do pretty well these days, but I have rarely ever felt well. My doctor told me that, when I am on, I knock the ball right out of the park. And then, something funny about me, I stand there and look behind me and say, where'd it go?

"Aren't you rather unassuming, Jane?" I laugh.

Dr. Dobbins, there's way more to come. I was trying to get into medical school. I transferred to another huge university

49

where I could hike and run, University of Utah. I did pretty well.
Still heavy and sluggish, though, but I had some room to
play...with food. I read medical journals a lot, and I manipulated
protein intake. Everything was reduced down to amino acids and
neurotransmitters. I did pretty well my junior year. I stayed in
the dorm, but I stayed to myself. Got really good grades,
somehow. Sleep was still a big issue for me. I guess it'll always be
a bit too much to handle.

I knew that I also had trouble with language. I was beyond
creative, if you'd even call it that. And I kept drifting farther and
farther out there, one planet at a time. My senior year, I tried
moving into an apartment. I stalled when trying to sign leases,
just couldn't make the connection, couldn't understand the lease,
fine print did me in. I slept in my car for over a year, sometimes
with the motor running and the heat on. Or under the stars. And
I drove everywhere.

In my life today, sleeping under a bridge doesn't frighten
me. Cardboard doesn't make me jump. I have hugged so many
mattresses, foam rubber pads, blankets, chairs. It didn't matter, I
couldn't sleep. Every little noise made me jump or drive
somewhere else. And you know, I never knew if those noises were
real or not. I wore the same sweat clothes for a year, sometimes a
coat. If I needed a bath, I'd wait for it to rain! It was so cool!

Jane's quiet, and I don't want to hear all of this. Not
because I'm annoyed, but because I find myself hurting for
her. Would I have walked by if I saw her in college? My
shame hit me hard.

"Did you have any friends?"

Emily Dickinson, Jeremiah Johnson, Harriet Tubman, Abe
Lincoln, Anne Frank, to name a few. Well, there was actually a
graduate student in clinical psychology. He was nice to me. He
asked me if I ever felt as if I had bugs crawling under my skin. I

told him not all the time. He said, "Goddam, goddam, you are so goddam strong!" I didn't know what on earth that was all about. I never saw him again. Oh well.

I didn't tell you about the time I was getting ready to actually take a bath at my parents' home when I saw a praying mantis by the drain. I thought, Wow. I went to get a bowl to put it in and take it outside. I got distracted, as usual, and when I went back to get it, there were all kinds of babies in there, too. Wow, I thought, amazing! Well, I ran and got the Polaroid and took pictures of them all. Then I put them outside. I made several trips. I then thought, oh my, what if they don't show up in the pictures, you know? I was praying they would, and they were praying, too! Well, it was a miracle that this happened to me, so cool, and a miracle they were real. I didn't want a picture of just a bath tub, you know?

Dr. Dobbins muffles a laugh.

Oh, you were asking about friends...then there was this lawyer guy, I guess he was a friend, who told me to lay off the cocaine. I wasn't doing any cocaine, and I realized I needed to keep that to myself. I just went along with it, like o-kaaaay.

When I took Abnormal Psychology, I realized that I needed to stay under cover. I was scared to death of getting locked up in some long-term, state institution. It hit me smack in the face that this would likely be my destiny. Somewhere in me, I knew that I should get the prize, the best mattress in some state hospital. Thorazine Shuffle is not exactly the jitterbug, you know?

"So, Jane, part of you knew you were dealing with a big problem."

Jane gets serious.

I think it went a bit beyond an attitude, and I didn't have much luck, dumb or what have you. I had one foot in denial and

51

one foot on the run. I literally tried to outdo my symptoms. Don't ask me how. I would drive, run, hide, and study some. Study, ha! I always had the radio blasting, because it was driving me nuts to hear voices. I'd also exercise myself into exhaustion, too. I do sleep better when I exercise.

My junior year, I did a research study in a sociology class. I asked students if they'd rather have terminal cancer or schizophrenia. They all said terminal cancer. All of them, every darn one of them. I said why. They said because people are mean to mentally ill people and that they wouldn't know what was happening to them. Yes, I knew I was in big trouble. So I thought I could fake it. Only thing is that I would always know and would always suffer and felt like I would likely die soon.

Like I'd be standing on a curb and get run over by a bus. Or someone would see my illness in me and would shoot me. However, everyone pretty much scattered if I did something insane, like passing out fliers that said help the mentally ill, trying to set up an underground to protect the mentally ill, you know, like runaway slaves, where's it safe for us to be in this society. People would just stare and walk away. Was it something I said? I'd ask. No, it was everything I did, I'd answer. Always talking to myself. I seriously never remember studying. Even in high school, I was always doing something else.

Okay, I realized that radio waves weren't being broadcasted through the fillings in my teeth. Good, right? However, my thoughts were blaring out of street lamps, they looked like speakers to me, so I would cover my ears and run. Oh man, everyone except me knows what I'm thinking! I knew I needed to stop that shit if I was going to be a physician. Know what I mean?

I'm sure my mouth was dropped open. Jane kept right on talking.

And I was driving myself nuts, stepping in pot holes,
thinking I'd blow the whole city up. I was scared out of my mind
that someone would get hurt by my stepping in pot holes. I tried
not stepping in them, as if they were land mines, and it gave me
headaches. All of my thoughts were painted against the sky, and it
stormed anything but rain, colors, colors, but no rainbows. It felt
like a huge war zone. It all felt so real.

Somehow I took graduate school entrance exams.
Somehow I showed up in the right lecture hall with a number 2
pencil, which they passed out anyway. There was this one
classmate sitting for one of the exams, and she was crying before
we even took the test, can you believe it? I told her to grab a
pencil and get a grip, you know, get a grip, girl!

My biggest problem, on the other hand, was figuring out
how to get home to see my sister graduate from college. How
could I go without getting caught? I always had this horrifying
nightmare of a dog catcher after me. To me, it paralleled exactly
what was going on in true life. I showed up at my parents' home,
though, wearing sweat clothes, a bandana, sunglasses, and a
walkman blasting a tape of The Who. I wore that tape out.

I don't exactly remember how I got home, I think by plane.
I guess I got on the right one, which I haven't always done.
(You'd think they'd check your ticket.) I sure as heck remember
being there. It was not fun, as if anything ever had been for years.
I couldn't do anything right. Where does our society get all these
rules, like we memorize them, when? And we just, duh, do
everything without any thought whatsoever? Apparently so. I
will always be disturbed, I wager, complaining about one thing or
another. There's much work that needs doing, Dr. Dobbins.

Jane kind of laughs, as if providing herself with a
moment of self-relief.

I really shouldn't be laughing at myself. It's not funny.

53

Not funny at all. I make myself nervous at times. I'm trying to figure out how the heck I made it – man, where was home, what was my future, who was going to be mad at me, where do you put people like me, and it's constant, always will be, and I guess I accept that. I just do. What choice do I have, I'd like to know.

I sit quietly and listen. There is a tremendous pause, and I'm thinking I've heard of this kind of disorder but have never seen a person with it. Jane grabs hold of some composure and comes back to our time, this time, the present. We're two people, and I don't know how to help. Jane looks up at me and says not to worry, it does no one any good. Oh man, she *rescued* me. And *I'm* the therapist.

I'll write this next part. For now, I need to go. I feel like I'm going to explode. It's traumatic for me to even tell you what happened. People have no clue what they take for granted. Do you?

I just look at Jane, dumbfounded. I'm there for her if only to listen. She smiles a tired and heavy smile. I ask her if she can trust me to lean on. She mumbles how frightening. Damn! Then she tells me it's time. Time for what? I ask, hoping she feels there's some help in me. Time to go, she says, and she's gone. I feel so small. She has such a wide consciousness, and I often feel left in the dark. How does she go about forgiving so many people? How has she gotten a grip? What am I doing? I've never felt like such an idiot.

I swing by to see my parents. My mother asks me to vacuum. The vacuum cleaner is too heavy, she says. It's the same it's always weighed, and I feel sad. Of course I'll vacuum, I tell her.

Being a good parent is a tough job because it never ends. At some point, the kids can take control and give love

54

in return. There is always a bond and an energy that waits to be fulfilled. It can be a hug or saying I love you or thank you. It means saying what you need to tell them, as if it's the last time you might see them. That's how forgiveness works for Jane. She writes and sends me the following:

I do remember getting on a plane to go home. I try to contain myself. We drive to my sister's college. Everyone's appalled at my dress code. No, everyone gapes. My mother hands me a dress to wear. I think I'm going to die. I think they wish I would.

My mother has a run in her hose. She tells me to drive to a drug store and buy her more hose. I get totally turned around and completely lost and make us late. My parents rant and rave, telling me I'm going to ruin my sister's graduation. I, myself, think I'm a miracle for even trying to get there. Damn, I'm tired of this getting-in-the-way-of-people's-lives feeling. Ridiculous. What's more ridiculous is having to change into a dress while we're in the car and on our way to campus.

My parents carry on and on about 'my behavior' and, following the ceremony, make me stay in the motel room while everyone else goes to dinner. I lie on the bed, my head spinning. I cry profusely. I am so far gone, and no one cares. The bed is spinning, and I go in the bathroom and bawl my eyes out. I don't sleep at all, but I go back and lie on the bed and dare not move, even when my family returns. I'm scared to death of the ruining things issue. I want to run away. But there's got to be someone who cares. I even thumb through the Yellow Pages and think to myself, who is apparently the only one connected to me, that this is awful. I'm just filled to the brim with shame and complete disbelief over 'me'.

It's morning, and we head for home. We stop to eat lunch. I go through the motions, not really able to pay attention to the process of ordering food. I get a taco salad, a cheeseburger, large fries, chili, a shake, a coke and...My dad says whoa and then asks me why so much food. I'm trying to stay grounded, I whisper. He says nothing more.

We drive home in silence, The Who blasting through my brain. I go to my room and flop on the bed. My dad won't let me go outside, even if only to wander around the neighborhood for an outlet. I sit quietly except for The Who, as I try to learn how not to stir. My dad comes in my room and says, Jane, I have Dr. Jobson on the phone, will you talk with him? Well, why are you asking me, Dad, I didn't call him, I say sweetly. Too confusing for me, I'm thinking. Please, will you come and just talk with him, my dad pleads. Somehow I feel very bad for my dad, and I stumble to the phone.

Oh no, I say to Dr. Jobson, not the hospital. I'm dead in the water, but I go. It's all over for me.

My dad and I walk in and ride the elevator to the psychiatric floor. Dr. Jobson is waiting for us. He says, Welcome back to earth. I tell him, What a dumb thing to say. Where's earth, I ask. He chats with my dad, just petty stuff, which annoys me to no end. Then my dad tells him 'everything' I had done...Excuse me? I say. I correct his grammar every chance I get. Seems like my only defense.

Dr. Jobson says he has more information now. And why not before, I ask. I understand more of what you go through now, he says. I look at Dr Jobson. I look at my dad. And I'm very quiet, but I'm thinking I'll never ride another elevator in my life.

I follow a nurse to a room and hug one of the countless mattresses I cling to in my pathetic life. I'm caught. There goes every ounce of my freedom for-ever. My dad rats me out, dumps me there and just leaves.

I fight my diagnosis, not wanting to be labeled

56

*schizophrenic. I plead with Dr. Jobson, knowing that my brain is
filled with holes and lesions. Actually, I believe that it's Multiple
Sclerosis, I say, I know it's MS. I can feel it, some unknown agent
gnawing at my mind, my heart and my soul. It's for real, I holler,
refusing to take any medication until I see a neurologist.*

*I meet a younger man who has black, curly hair. I am
sitting on an exam table, my feet dangling over the edge as I
wiggle my toes and concentrate on answering his questions. He
asks me if I hear voices. Right then, a page comes over the
intercom from the ceiling. I feel confused by this and say, I heard
that, did you? A vein pops out of his forehead, and he clenches his
fists. I sit, waiting for an answer. Goddam schizophrenics, he
says, and stomps out of the room. Dr. Jobson comes in several
minutes later, and sheepishly, with my head hanging very low, I
tell him I think I've been diagnosed. There is no more mention of
MS or schizophrenia. I still wonder if he heard the page.*

*I'm back in my room, and a nurse gives me some meds. A
social worker comes in and tells me to come to group. She's nice
but too pushy for me. Get real, I tell her, go save some other
world. I try to make it to group, and it takes me five days before
I'm actually sitting there with some clue of what's going on.*

*Today, it's a psychiatrist leading the group. Two
thousand years ago, Jesus walked on this earth, he recites. He is
soon due to return, he says. It's silent for a long time. No one
seems to think they're Jesus, I say, except maybe do you? I was
very confused by that whole ordeal.*

*I'm feeling more social, and I venture to the nurse's
station. Hi, I say, which one of you is St. Mary? They all stop
what they're doing and stare at me. Then the social worker smiles
and says "No, honey, St. Mary's is just the name of the hospital."
They laugh. Oh, I say, totally confused. I decide to walk around.*

After a long while of walking in the circular unit with

hallways branching out, that same social worker says, "My, you're getting some exercise!" I say, no, I'm just trying to find my room, any ideas? Inpatient provides some difficulties. I keep trying. She points down a hallway, and I say thank you. She's very nice.

What can I say about my parents? My dad feels like a terrible parent for not knowing sooner what had been going on with me, like, a doctor's daughter living out of her car for over a year. I told Dad not to worry about it, that I have storage space and a friend's couch at times, and that I wouldn't tell anyone. I guess I kind of graduated into my actual diagnosis, which was no picnic. You can't know something until it happens, I tell my dad. You picked up on what's there and called Jobson, and you can't really diagnose someone over the phone very well, I say. Oh, I give up, he's just going to feel responsible for things he's not responsible for. How do you tell someone it isn't his or her fault? You can't with him. Fine.

My mother is the one who is really hurting. She comes to visit after I've been in the hospital a few days. She looks as if she's about ready to die of guilt and sadness. Here's the stupid thing she says: Jane, I am so sorry. I tried to be a good mother. Here's what I say to her: Mom, for crying out loud, you didn't do this.

I hurt terribly for her. I'm fuming over psychological theories but say nothing. I give my mom a hug.

Dr. Jobson has me on a neuroleptic, which is an antipsychotic, plus lithium. The meds make me feel slow. I'm groggy, trouble focusing and making connections, colors everywhere. Maybe it's been for me like being on LSD without being on it. Nonetheless, Dr. Jobson tells me I'm getting better. Oh, okay, I'm not seeing it, I say. To me, it seems as if my brain is rewinding. Okay, I say again, I don't know what to think. Or how to think. I avoid any discussion about my diagnosis. It's as if

58

I need to be in denial about what I'm truly up against. It's better for me to just know my symptoms, such as insomnia, hallucinations, delusions. I start counting on the meds to put a dent in the symptoms. I don't know that I can make real friends. It's scarey. I grieve over the loss of my friends who had been dead a good while anyway.

After two weeks, Dr. Jobson lets me go. I realize that they aren't going to lock me up forever. It would have been nice if I'd known that, but I know deep down that there's still a terminal bed for me in some back ward. My dad drives me home, and I ask him what I can and can't do. He says, what do you mean? I say, Can I get the mail? Can I jump on the trampoline? He asks me, why not? I say, Dad, I'm a mental patient. I'm on an antipsychotic medication. I'm supposed to sit in a rocking chair, if I can even pull that off. And oh man, what will the neighbors think? Don't worry about the neighbors, he says. Hmm. Okay, I say, but I am going to quote you, Dad.

Hey, howdy neighbor, we're not supposed to worry about you! Who cares. Aren't neighbors supposed to care? What if they don't get it? I stay close to home for a few days, not sure what to do or say. I have started sleeping, which is a new thing. I guess it's my symptoms that have kept me awake, like a front row seat at a horror movie or a kaleidoscope.

My test scores for both medical school and graduate school arrive in the mail. On the same day, can you believe it? I look at my scores and decide they're all a mistake. I show them to my parents. Applying to medical school is a go; my scores are up there. And my graduate school scores are in the 97th percentile. My parents are really trying hard to figure out how I pulled that off. Actually, they just sit there, as they often haven't a clue what to do or say.

I also find out that, even though I finished my final

semester, I am three credits short of graduating from college. You'd think I could somewhat count, but I guess I missed that one. I whip through a correspondence course, but there's no graduation ceremony for me. God or someone never really put things as such on my schedule.

It's one week after I'm discharged from the hospital, and I decide I need a job. Dad told me not to worry about a bunch of things. He's in denial, thinking I'm mild bipolar or something totally off base, but it works for me. I go back to St. Mary's and run into the graduate student who assessed me. She says hi. I tell her I made it out somehow but shh, not to tell anyone. She laughs and says okay. I say, yeah, I even gave Nurse Ratched a hug. I tell her I'm looking for a job. She says "Jesus" under her breath. I say, he's running group.

She laughs again, then pauses and says, you go, girl. I think to myself, did she learn that in graduate school? No, she learned that from me when she was fumbling around with those ink blot cards. I said, Hey, I don't care if they're not in order, and I won't tell your professor, you just go, girl! I bet I had the most far-out answers on every one of those tests that day. The rings of Saturn! That's a long ways off.

There are no jobs. I go to another hospital. I get a job as an orderly. I wheel patients around. I'm careful pushing someone on a stretcher, and my brain says, yee-haw! I'm not going to let things get to me, and I try not to take myself too seriously. I have fun on the job, doing well with the patients, but it's never glitch-free. One morning, I wake up, and I swear to God, I'm thinking there's a tidal wave coming. Get to the post office, I holler to my parents.

They convince me to get in the car, which is no easy doing. Get in the car. Get in the car! Get in the bleeping car! Okay, you don't have to say it like that. Maybe you do. We drive to the hospital in silence. We are driving to where I work. I figure we'll go to the top floor, which incidentally is the psychiatric unit. I tell my parents to hurry, hurry! We go in a room and sit. I don't want to sit. Dr. Jobson walks in. What's up, he asks. I look at him and, only then, but miraculously, I catch on to what's happening. Help me, I say, I'm disconnected.

CHAPTER SIX DISCONNECTED

Does anyone bring mental patients flowers when they're in the hospital, that's *the big deal.*

Dr. Jobson says okay, and I try to tell him what I'm thinking. Emotionally, it's excruciating for me. Literally, I believe that the two halves of my brain have burst apart at the corpus collosum and are suspended in air above my head, attached with two wires. I pull my hair and just want to scream, but I don't. We've got to get milk for the kids, I then say, they're malnourished. Stay away from the windows, we're about to be hit, I say with utter concern. I experience myself in an array of altruistic delusions.

The pain is real to me, and it's killing me to know that people in this world need help. Can anyone understand this? I am stuck between asleep and awake, and I am at the world's mercy.

Dr. Jobson ups my meds and sends me home. I clutch the bedpost in my room, still thinking I'm on a raft, having survived the tidal wave. My dad tries to check on me, and I tell him not to walk in, that my soul has fallen out and is somewhere on the floor. He looks upset. Look, just give me some time, I tell him.

A few mornings later, it's Saturday. I wake up, run in the kitchen and holler at my mom: The Redcoats are coming, and they all have guns! She tells me to go back to bed and to try getting up again. I do that. I run in the kitchen again and tell her they're gone. She says, good. We pause. Then I say, you don't happen to know which way they went, do you? Jane, please...Okay, Mom, I'll go back to bed. She reaches exasperation readily, and I learn from her what cues are.

Sometimes I can't tell what's real. I'm real, that's for sure. My disorder is real, I know that. And to me, it feels very chemical. So I adjust to a higher dosage, and I go back to work. I don't know if the hospital employees know that I saw my doctor in the very hospital where I work. I still have my job, and I will never know who knows what. Some of the other orderlies make cracks about 'schizophrenics'. I ask Dr. Jobson if he knows if they know. He doesn't know either, and he's smart. So I decide not to worry about it.

He says to me, "They may know. They may not know." I learn to use that in tolerating ambiguity and then moving forward, as if some things cannot possibly matter. I then tell myself, they may matter; they may not matter. And then I move forward. Looking back, I'd say I've survived monstrous uncertainties.

I work as an orderly for a year and then pack up to go to medical school at University of Tennessee in Memphis. It seems I reached a point of being afraid of being too far away from home, like in the Rockies, or Northeast. I define my disorder as follows: sick, well, and in-between. And there are a whole lot of symptoms, some that became very obvious in college. Looking back, you think! I just try to stay on track, and I find myself dissecting a cadaver. I smell that awful smell, and I wonder what kind of a life this guy had. Some medical students are eating their lunch, chicken sandwiches. God, I hope they don't get mixed up.

I feel connected to my cadaver in a kindred-spirit way. I say that because I'm told that the cadavers come from homeless people who have died. And since I've been homeless, I'm wondering, if I suddenly discovered I knew this guy, what then? I met all kinds of people when I was living out of my car. Phew!

I live in student housing, and I am studying bones, learning the names. It reminds me of breaking both legs, ripping apart my knee and destroying my ankle when competing as a teenager. Teenager, teenager, where has my life gone? Was there not another road I could have taken? Are some things just etched in stone? I swear, I could be a better adult if I were just twelve all the time.

I try to sleep, and I feel a bright light above me, like an operating room. It dawns on me that medical school, being a physician, is going to mess with my sleep, and vice versa. You'd think I would have known that. I close my eyes and see body parts falling out of people's skin. I smell formaldehyde and wonder if it's an olfactory hallucination. No, it's coming from my finger tips.

Night after night, I get up and pace the small space by my bed. I realize that I can't do this. I hang in there a long while, but I'm genuinely afraid that I'll get into that disconnected place and have no help. I go talk with the dean after just a few months in medical school. I withdraw, saying that I have an illness that has come back. Knowing when to fold in poker, how important is it to know how to do that: VERY.

My parents are upset, and it feels as if they are upset with me. It's simply that they don't know what to do, but I do. There's always another hand to draw, I tell myself, as I set my cards down on the table. I tell them to please not worry, that I'll work something out. My mom says, what are you going to do with your life? She seems exasperated.

I'm thinking about addressing some of my symptoms, getting a job that will force me to talk, I say. Communication trouble is an issue I need to face head on. Then maybe I'll see about graduate school in psychology. I do know that if I'm going to be a psychologist, I've got to learn to talk. I've got to stop having to practice what to say in my mind prior to...and I've also got to learn to keep my mouth shut when best. Sometimes that just seems impossible, but I'll give it a go.

I'm hired as a server at a small restaurant. I come across

as relaxed and confident, using the strategy of faking it 'til I make it. Underneath, there's a rumbling in my soul, and I wonder where my life's going. I get through moment by moment at the restaurant. One server was doing drugs with his brother and stabbed him to death. I was overwhelmed with horrendous sadness. How on earth...

One night, before I serve my last customers, the manager tells me to get the mop, cleaner, rubber gloves...and clean the restrooms. That means I'll be walking right by my customers. It occurs to me that he's doing this to save himself a few pennies on my time card. I tell him no. He says if I don't, I'm fired. I say, no, I quit.

I'm driving home, worrying about what to tell my parents. I tell them nothing, not wanting to face their anxiety. I know that when a door closes, look for a window. That's just how I operate, you know, common sense and trying to do the right things. What's available for me? It's a search.

Within days, I find a big, fancy restaurant that's hiring. The manager asks me if I've ever served tables. I say, about eleven. He laughs. How I get the job, I don't know. So I ask why he's hired me. He says he likes my smile. I think, what have I gotten myself into? Not knowing helps.

I have no clue how to cook at the patrons' tables: steak diane, steak cordon bleu, shrimp scampi, bananas foster, cherries jubilee and flaming drinks. I just pull my hair back when I have to make a flaming drink. They're tricky. I wear a tuxedo and turn on a smile. It's all I have at times.

I manage to catch on, and everything about me improves. I get to where I can serve a party of forty, knowing all of their drinks by memory. I learn, as many times over in my life, that I am the exception to rules. I love my job and am thinking I might be a server forever. I like it better than changing sheets on beds.

Wow, I've come a long way!

The manager tells me that the customers are always right. Even when they're wrong, they're right. How does that work? I take an order for hamburgers and bring two women their food. They complain, saying they ordered prime rib. They insist on prime rib for the price of the burgers. I go get the manager. I am certain they'll get prime rib and the burgers, all on my watch. Plus I bet I'll end up paying for their undeserved food with my tip money.

They tell the manager that I got the order wrong. Prepared to take a beating, I just stand there. The manager asks me what they ordered. I tell him the burgers. He tells the women that they need to leave. I walk away. I ask him later why he did that if the customers are always right. He tells me two things about myself: that I don't lie, and I say so if I make a mistake. I say to him, well, that's true.

Other interesting things happen to me at this restaurant. A guy leaves his motel key under my tip tray, and I holler at him across the restaurant. Hey, you might need this! I was holding up his key before I realized what was up with that. I got a ton of tips that night, and everyone thought I was hilarious. I am an expert when it comes to embarrassing myself, probably the best.

I develop my reflexes and stamina on the job. The other servers are fast. I try to keep up. They also wipe their noses a lot. I finally figure out that they snort cocaine, so I just say, wipe your nose. I ask them why they use cocaine. They say because it's a stressful job. I say cut back on your hours. They say no, they need the money. Why? I ask. They say to buy cocaine. I work like heck to be a team player, but it's just crazy. They make so many mistakes with orders.

I apply to graduate schools in psychology. I get to pick top name schools in the country, on account of my test scores. I miss competing, but not everything about traveling. One time, a guy showed me a condom. They make great water balloons, I say and walk off. I mean, he was so tacky.

Back when I was 15 years old, this guy in his late twenties came to my motel door at around 11:00 p.m. He showed me a condom, too – what is it with showing girls condoms, that it's romantic? This guy that woke me up at 11:00 p.m. was just over the top. I hollered at him really loud, "Does your mother know you're out this late?"

See, when I'm on, I really do knock the ball out of the park. Yet it is such an innocent thing, a surprising thing for me. My parents don't understand how it is that, if I get sent flowers for doing a great job, it jolts me. I'm not sure how to explain that, and my parents don't understand. I try to tell them I'm not used to such kinds of luxuries, and they just stare at me. Flowers, they ask? What's the big deal about flowers? Does anyone bring mental patients flowers when they're in the hospital, that's the big deal. Never sent me any. Did when I broke my leg, broke my ankle, ripped up my knee...Anyway, flowers are a huge deal, for me they are. That's one thing.

The other thing is that with my chemistry...it's just when the unexpected happens in a, I guess, good way - it trips me out, but I'll work on it. I'll get over it, but it's going to take some doing and undoing. Flowers will always be a huge deal, but I'll try to keep the shock wave from ripping through my nerves. Everyone happy now?

My dad sees that I'm serious about graduate school. He suggests I stay in town and go to graduate school there so he can keep an eye on me. I tell him, no, I've got to deal with this on my own. And I want a top name school. I want to be with the best and the smartest. My dad gets nowhere with me. Vanderbilt University, it is.

My mom and I drive to my new surroundings of Nashville and find an efficiency apartment. It's within walking distance of campus. I'm a three-hour drive from my parents. This feels good. I'm so excited, but can I cut it? Graduate school provides a bit more flexibility for me to wrap my sleep problems around my schedule, or vice versa, than a career in medicine.

My efficiency is like a mansion. I am so happy. My anxiety is as high as the ceiling; it's one of those fancy, very high ceilings. I am scared to death of flunking out. I am scared of my symptoms, because I never really know if I have control. I'm always having to check on myself and keep an eye on me. It gets old.

So all through my story, Dr. Dobbins, I am learning. So when I hear about what someone has done for me or compliments me or sends flowers, I just smile and say thank you. And any recognition? Smile and say thank you, I tell myself, ready to bust and wondering what's with my lithium level. It'll be okay. I can ease into some new reality if needed.

No one says it's easy to be an exception who wants only to follow the rules. The thing is, my disorder is something that certain, very special, other people have, too. There are many, and I wish I could be their voice. Don't consider my illness to be who I am. Or what other people are.

Just be kind to us and be patient. Send flowers on any occasion; celebrate life and be in it. Gather your courage and be of help. Don't shame us or bind us. We all have our difficulties. And trust me, I am so grateful for the help I have received, seriously. Yet, it's a burden. It's a terrible burden to connect with people at times. And the expectations on me of being a doctor's daughter have been excruciating. As for my illness, well, it's that 'elephant in the living room' ordeal. You know what I mean, everyone sees it, but no one says anything. Most of our family friends have never understood, anyway. I've usually just felt really stupid and incapable.

What gives me strength and hope is knowing that there really are many people who have elegant minds that we fail to treasure. They are rooting for me to knock the ball out of the park whenever I go to bat, even if no one else hears their cheers the way I do. My pain directs me, as does my disorder, and I love the mentally ill, even those I've never met. They are my heroes.

I think of those who were locked away or who have died, and I grit my teeth and tell myself that I am going to make things right. The people who killed themselves, who were locked up – if they can endure their pain or take their life, I can sure as heck help get our society where it should be.

***

I think of being a child, at age 5. The mother of two next-door neighbor boys slit her wrists. My dad found her in her bath tub. I remember some feeling of compassion I had for her and her family, and why? I kept asking. My life went on as normal, but their family was interrupted, with no going back.

I remember in 7th grade when my science teacher got very angry one day and walked out. He never came back. A few weeks later, I heard another teacher talking about him. She said he had a nervous breakdown. Nerves break? I wondered. What happened to him?

And another teacher left for the same reason, and another and another.

In 8th grade, a guy in my class told me his depression was killing him. I followed him everywhere, and he finally told me that, when he was six years old, his parents killed themselves, together. I cried.

In high school, there was a math teacher who laughed and cried and laughed and cried. He was fired. A year later, he came back to school dressed as Dracula, wanting to apply for the principal's job. He was escorted off the premises.

A coach I knew when I was sixteen years old was fired, and he killed himself.

A friend of mine in high school stopped coming to school and wouldn't come out of his room. Rumor had it that he developed schizophrenia. Everyone was quiet, and I never saw him again. I always wondered, but I never knew what happened to him.

A guy I met in college, who was absolutely brilliant, put a bullet through his head. Gone from here forever.

And these passing accounts are only a few. It made me realize that mental illness is everywhere. It's frightening for those who have them. It's frightening for those who don't. So aren't we all in the same boat? A shrimp boat no less, and shouldn't we all try to be more like Forrest Gump...life can be good. It's there for us, look and see clearly...if we'd just help each other.

CHAPTER SEVEN GRADUATE SCHOOL

I have always felt my presence in my soul.

August 21, 2009

I've been carried into a world that no one explained to me in graduate school. I learned very little about major, persistent and severe mental illness in my training. Jane is trying to open up to me. I feel a stillness in her voice, an occasional tremor, and a sincerity beyond words. She's often intense, exceedingly altruistic and filled with passion. She's trying to live for a cause, not die for one. Can you blame her? What else is she supposed to do? She asks me that.

In her undying efforts, she has no home, no kids to raise, no 'friends' who truly stand by her, always having a disorder that keeps her from sticking with a career, a job, one place to live, continuity, joy, success – oh, the list goes on forever, it seems. Her basic upkeep includes not caring about her hair or clothes unless she's trying to imitate others, to fit in. One time, she told me she always has so much else going on that she forgets appearances. She asked me about clothes: how is it decided what matches what? I had to tell her I don't really know. So then she started not worrying about it and would show up for sessions in colored toe socks and sandals. I can't help but both laugh and feel blessed to know her.

I have friends, and I go out with people. I've never been the type to marry or have kids. Both my clients and friends are important to me, and I'm happy single. I need nothing more. Yet I'm always open to people. So this is me, keeping it simple and enjoying the peace in my life. I love my private practice and my suite-mates. I love my clients of all ages.

Jane's struggles are hers. I feel content just listening and showing interest. I fear getting in the way of her process, and yet I get a bit annoyed at times. I think it's because she points out the limits of therapists, and I take it personally. It's all like a game of chess with her, and I try to concentrate on making the right move when it is my turn to do so. Jane has taught me about precision. I wish she could experience some fun with her genius. And I wish her anxiety would flatten right out. More than anything, I wish she could sleep with some continuity and peace.

She keeps pouring her heart out to me:

So where am I, at 25 years old? It's my first semester of graduate school. I feel nervous and scared. I write papers and take tests. I'm so shy. I worry that people will find out about me and will flunk me out. People like me shouldn't be psychologists, according to some. I need to hurry and get my PhD.

I have my master's thesis completed in six months. Phew! I have everything paid for by a National Insititute of Mental Health (NIMH) scholarship for four years. I'm wrong; it is up after one year. There's no way I can pay for tuition. And I have living expenses. I feel dead in the water. So I decide to walk around campus, just to be grateful for what I experience. Something will work out the way it's supposed to.

I have always felt my presence in my soul, my center. I've never understood the reason I'm made to suffer the way I do. Some of it is because of people. My actual disorder, though, doesn't have to be the total nightmare that it is. People's fears, misunderstandings and misconceptions have been very difficult in ways beyond the actual symptoms and efforts to make my disorder workable. I have worked and struggled in ways even I who live it cannot comprehend. Yes, people have ripped my heart out with their rude comments about the mentally ill, and they're going to become psychologists? It's compassion that keeps me going.

It's love that conquers all evil. It's love that makes the difference. It's our choices that allow us to love. It's our courage that helps us step up to the plate. Sometimes I think I am beautiful even when I am disordered – because of who I try so hard to be. I try so hard to do my best when I don't stand a chance. It's that I try anyway. If it were possible, I might walk away, but where would I go?

So I'm walking around campus, teary-eyed but grateful, when I run into a professor. He stops to talk, and I tell him my problem. He suggests I apply for a Clinical Fellowship at a practicum site that provides outpatient services. He says it's very competitive, but to try for it. It would pay my tuition. The Fellowship, I find out, is for two years. Well, that'll do for now, I tell myself, and I apply. Many students apply, but I'm in!

During my time there, I grow tremendously. It is still a time when I experience some scattered thoughts, disrupted sleep and trouble expressing my thoughts verbally. I deal with it successfully. Others wouldn't connect these symptoms to my disorder, but I do. However, I'm not any more "psychotic" than other graduate students, blending right in and acquiring a respect that I cannot fathom. I'm told I'm brilliant, and I just shrug my shoulders and say, what's up with that?

I get the toughest cases, and that comes by sheer accident. My clients' lives are reflected in a pile of leftover charts for us graduate students to choose from. Well, I don't have a choice, as I stand there wondering what this exercise is all about. Finally, I scoop the "bottom of the barrel" file folders up in my arms and walk to my office. I see that all eight of my clients-to-be have the *diagnosis of Borderline Personality.*

It's written in bold red print on page one. Can't miss it. I soon find out why my peers scurry while looking through the charts. My supervisor wants me to swap some of my charts with the other students. She says that these clients can be the toughest to work with. Of course, that further piques my interest, and I tell her I'd like to give it a go. They are people, aren't they, I ask. They can get better, I'm sure, I say. She says that I'd better be on top of it. What for, I ask. For your sake, she says. Hmm.

My supervisor tells me a story about a woman who has Borderline Personality Disorder. This woman stopped seeing her therapist but would drive by his office every day and feel relieved from seeing his car. So one day, she ended up in a psych unit. It turned out her therapist bought a new car. This is a problem unlike mine, but that poor woman, I'm thinking, someone needs to help her. I tell my supervisor that this woman's therapist really failed her, that he should have helped her stay connected to herself or something she owns that reminds her of her goodness or her worth or something besides him, not him. We kick around this idea a bit, and she says I am going to be an excellent therapist.

So here I am working 30 clinical hours with BPD clients whom I consider amazing challenges and who get better! I also am awarded a 20-hour research assistanceship. I'm carrying a full load of classes, and I also have oral exams, a dissertation, and everything else. After two years, my Fellowship is up, and the director grants me two more years. I don't think that's ever been done, if so, rarely. I earn a stellar reputation. I also experience grave losses during that time. My grandparents die. My major adviser dies. My best friend dies.

I stay on the lithium and antipsychotic medication. Of course, I just roll with it. I have no idea that the most demanding symptoms are simmering right below the surface. I take one day at a time. I thrive on developing clinical skills. I present papers at national conferences. I continue to be clueless; for example, why am I the only student, among all these professors, presenting a paper? Oh, so that's what a symposium is...I was the only student on the panel, and I bet this is just normal. Maybe. Maybe not. I do well answering the questions from the audience.

I realize the hardships that some of my relatives have endured. Many seemed troubled, some just eking out an existence. I feel guilty, sad and undeserving. Why should I have a better life? Is my life better? Shouldn't my parents have known about genetics sooner and opted, safely, not to have kids? Graduate school provides me with somewhat of a distraction from my disorder. Seems so. Or I'm just lucky. I think much of it has to do with having control of my schedule, the freedom to take care of me, doing what I need to do when I need to and working very hard. It is paradise.

I put the papers down and take a deep breath. I had no idea that she went this far with her education, although I knew she was incredibly smart. Intelligence and education, however, are two different things. So she's both educated and smart. And she has a monster of a disorder to contend with. How does she do it? And what the heck is she doing working as a tech at a treatment center?

Jane seems to be on a roll. She drops off more pages for me to read. Part of me wants to be caught up in her story, and part of me needs to feel grounded. She has an effect on me that I'm not sure how to explain. I feel ashamed at times for my own bias. Her story continues:

I've left some things out that I think are important. Dr. Jobson wanted me to see a psychologist when I was being discharged from my first psych unit. I was dead set against it. When I came back from medical school, he encouraged me again. I agreed to see someone. This was when I was working in the restaurant and applying to graduate schools. Well, it was a long drive to see this psychologist, but I was okay with that.

However, he laughed when I told him I was applying to clinical psychology programs. He laughed! He told me that I needed to see him three times per week, as in who would be paying for that? He told me that I'd make a good physician (just back from medical school, are you not listening), but that I didn't understand people. So true, he was an enigma to me! How can someone be so cruel...I was done. Except he said he was okay with a drug holiday, and back inpatient I went.

It doesn't end there. Jobson lined me up three more psychologists, none of whom did any better, and it occurred to me that they were all a bit freaked out by my diagnosis. Hello, there's a person in here, I'd say, waving my hand. That didn't help. So I finally told Dr. Jobson that I'd find someone on my own. I closed my eyes and picked my psychologist with my pointer finger running through the yellow pages. Yep, just like that ad — let your fingers do the walking...except I was in a hurry.

I told the psychologist not to call Dr. Jobson, that I simply wanted some help dealing with stress. I only saw him eight or nine times before it was time to move and start school, but he helped me a lot. He helped me feel like Jane, because that's me. There is normal in me somewhere; I call it the real me. He thought I could breeze through graduate school. I wouldn't say that, by any means, but I certainly appreciated his vote of confidence and encouragement. What he thought of as a breeze, I knew as a tornado. The point, though, is that I survived most of the harrying experiences any normal student would go through. It was the first significant leg of a long and winding, colorful journey in becoming a professional.

***

It's 1988, and I'm 28 years old. I've been seeing another psychologist throughout graduate school. He knows everything about me. He's terrific, caring and warm. The great thing about him is that he just completed graduate school, which maybe seems to allow him to be open and able to see me for me and not through a diagnostic manual that, it seems, one uses to stereotype. (What is my stereotype, because that I have never figured out.) As therapists age and grow, it seems that some of them get calloused and treat people more like a disorder instead of like people. He teaches me a lot about my strengths. I have great interest in understanding everyone's strengths. I'm not saying that I have succeeded, but people matter to me. I love hearing about people's own realities.

It's so interesting to me, being a therapist and also a client. I think to myself, whoa, what would it be like to see my therapist in blue jeans, grocery shopping? Do therapists really have lives? Do they have kids? Do they exist between sessions? Am I just a bit self-centered? I think sometimes that a therapist can be a higher power and exist 'just for my sake'. I think this allowed me to help myself gain some confidence and normalcy. And how do my clients see me? I don't know, they all say with great appreciation. That's good.

When it comes to my clients, I do find them tough nuts to crack. Borderline Personality Disorder is a diagnosis in a class of mental disorders very unlike my disorder. I don't have a personality disorder. I try to put my own disorder aside, and it allows me to be of great help to others unlike me. Yet aren't we all sort of 'out of order' in some way or another, just trying to survive? Different symptoms, but maybe still a similar pain, just expressed differently, and a need to accept oneself.

Don't we all face and endure difficulties that beckon us to reach for help in some sideways fashion, grasp for straws or become care-less at times? We should care more. Don't you think? Sometimes it's enough just to stay afloat. I see my clients as individuals with their own uniqueness and strengths. I really enjoy watching them improve. Boundaries keep them from wearing me out.

I take a look at my master's thesis again - attributions, responsibility and blame. I use up a whole lot of paper just getting down to the basic realization: most people blame victims for their problems. They find fault with victims in a way that distances them from becoming that victim. They say that's not me, never can be me. Deep down, though, we fear becoming a victim. So we tell ourselves lies. Maybe you get my point. But what is a victim? Am I a victim? Do I see myself as a victim? I'm not sure. I don't think I feel as such. Too busy trying to make it.

We are a society filled to the brim with fear of the unknown and prejudice. People want to feel safe and secure, it seems. I hope to impress upon you, Dr. Dobbins, how utterly frightening it is for me to be disordered in our society. You will see, I hope, as I continue my story. I'm surprised that I've not been killed, although it feels like death when people try to talk me out of my freedom.

And it's being assigned limits to me based on a diagnosis that leads me to run from those psychologists. Helping someone find limits is one thing. Defining what a client can and cannot do, based on a disorder's stereotype, is nothing short of playing God.

I also know that, only by luck or some huge power over us all, our culture has not thrown me away. Do I truly belong in a garbage heap? How can I be beautiful and brilliant one moment, valued and praised...and then, bang, game over in seconds? I know how that can happen. I know how I've gotten back on my feet, too, with a great difficulty that most people couldn't

78

imagine. Of course I know - I've lived it.

CHAPTER EIGHT GOING TO JAIL

I'm stalling and repeating myself; a reminder, as if I know something is going to happen.

I have my classes behind me. I'm in my fourth year in graduate school. My mom comes to visit, and I tell her how tired I am. I tell her that some days I hit a wall, smack, like a bug on a windshield. Only it's a wall; you'd think I'd see it. She understands enough to tell me that I always have a home with my dad and her – if I ever need that. I cry tears of relief and sorrow.

Other days, I find some inner strength that raises me up. I see myself as an adjunct professor with a part-time private practice. One supervisor who knows me well considers me one of the best therapists he has known. The faculty write recommendation letters for me to go on internship, one of them saying I'm one of the best students, if not the best...and the most intelligent person he knows in certain ways. I'm not a rocket scientist, thankfully, but I have a gift. I'm very good at understanding people and things. You know, actually, all of this is harder than rocket science, in my opinion.

My supervisors, after my first clinical year, tape record and videotape my sessions with clients to use as teaching devices. In my second year of clinical work, I am supervising students who are part of our practicum site eating disorders team. I'm not exactly sure what I do that sets me apart. However, people recognize it and are drawn to me. Whatever it is that people like, it's something about my personality.

I was loving and compassionate toward the mentally ill long before I became ill, and it feels almost as if I was born that way. One time, a retired physician said to me, "Now you listen *hard to this. I'm going to tell you something that I've rarely ever said. If someone doesn't like you, Jane, there's something wrong with that person." I just said, Hmm. There are a lot of things people say that I'm not sure I have ever fully understood. I may never.*

I'm a work-in-progress, a contradiction. I want to tear down the wall and show folks the myths, that's all they are – myths. My confusion is genuine and forthcoming, and I try to make sense of it.

So the strong help the weak in a better world, anyway. Change is everywhere. One minute, we're on top of the world. The next minute, who knows? When that happens and people scatter, find the nice people. Stick with them. They can grow in numbers if we simply play our cards right. In your marathon swim, find the islands (the good moments, the good people), Dr. Jobson encourages with a grim smile on his concerned face.

I'm stalling and repeating myself; a reminder, as if I know something is going to happen. Change. I tell Dr. Jobson that I'm going to stay put in Nashville indefinitely, meaning I wouldn't be driving the distance to see him every few months. He makes a referral, and I find myself sitting in another psychiatrist's office. I flip through a magazine, nervous and hopeful that he's good.

I follow him into a big room with a huge view of a park. He positions himself at his desk and motions for me to sit on a distant couch. I ignore his stiff manner, and we chat. I tell him about my symptoms, my history, my life. He tells me that there's no way I could be making it through graduate school with the disorder I'm describing – especially chronic and severe. I stop cold and think: Dr. Jobson told me he's never seen a case more severe. I know it's chronic because I know what I live with. What's up with this guy, denying my reality, arguing with me over the truth? You need to call Dr. Jobson, I say, pick up the phone.

81

He keeps making the case that what I'm doing can't be done. Hmm, maybe my struggles are over. He's also concerned about tardive dyskinesia, a side effect that can appear when taking antipsychotic medication. It involves the involuntary movements of one's lower jaw and tongue, facial tics, and so on. You see this side effect a lot in state mental hospitals with patients who have been on Thorazine most of their lives. Like at least one relative I know of. It's offensive, debilitating, intrusive and telling. I worry.

So agreed: a new reality that I'm just a little bipolar – the power of reason? A convincing commercial? The psychiatrist pulls me off the neuroleptic. I'm okay for just a bit. Then I literally capsize. I feel myself exiting my physical well-being. My boundaries of verbal expression dissipate. I am no longer the me that I need to be – to even somewhat make it in my life. Game over.

***

Symptoms continue to surface. It's late at night; the clock says 11:26. That's okay, because I feel like going for a jog. My boyfriend, Carl, is snoring. How I met Carl is a story of its own. We found ourselves meeting abruptly and needing one another at times when it really counted. This night, it's his turn to be there for me. I poke at him until he wakes up. Get up, come on, time to go, I say.

I pull on my sneakers. Carl and I have an understanding that, wherever I go, he tags along. Jesus, Carl, get up. Carl is very religious and, although sex outside of marriage is allowed, he tells me not to say Jesus like that. Carl is one who goes by the rules he chooses to go by.

I tell him to hurry. He gets up and jams his big feet in his cowboy boots. Put some pants on, for crying out loud, and don't lecture me about Jesus, I say. He pulls some over-sized sweat pants on. You want to go eat? he asks. No, we're going for a run,

I say impatiently. Jane, he says, not now. Come on, I say, and out the door I go.

Carl shifts gears and puts the leather to the pavement. He's running down the street, chasing me as I decide I'm going to run a marathon. I ran in the Boston Marathon when I was 16 years old, and I feel due for a repeat. In Carl's mind, he simply wants to be sure I'm safe. He also knows that I see a shrink.

I sprint for a mile and end up close to campus. Some woman on a set of stairs leading to an apartment sees me and Carl and yells for me to come up the stairs. It actually occurs to me that it's a domestic violence shelter. Except a cop pulls up right as I am trying to bolt up the stairs and tells me to stop. I stop, but I stand there, jumping up and down.

Carl catches up and bends over, with his hands on his knees, trying to catch his breath. The cop tells me he's taking me downtown. Great, I say with enthusiasm. Will you drive alongside me while I run? I ask him. He tells me to get in the car. Get in the car. Get in the car. Instead of swearing at me, the way my parents do, he cuffs me.

I didn't want Carl to feel left out, and that lady on the stairs was still standing there. He needs to go, too, I tell the cop. Right about then, another cop arrives on the scene. The cop asks me what Carl has done to me. He's spiritually abusive, lecturing me about Jesus. He's a hypocrite, that, too, I say, still jumping up and down and not yet in the car. So they stick him in the other car. Wow, we each have our own rides. Let's race!

Yet somehow this isn't right. They book me for public intoxication, and where's the beer? There's no beer and no drugs. I tell them, I don't even smoke pot! They say, yeah, we know that. I sit in a cell all alone. And that's when it dawns on me. I'm safe, but not safe. It partly occurs to me that this has to do with medication. Oh my. The guard tells me, after hours of being in jail, that they'll let me out – if I calm down. If that's true, I'll be in jail for my entire lifetime. This is not good.

Things become more difficult. They slide me food on a tray through a slot. I slide it back untouched. How can I be sure they aren't trying to poison me? I can't. I check out my cell. There's a bunk bed. I leap up and onto the top bunk. I lie there in the semi-darkness for about 27 seconds and hop down. I have to find a way to escape. I start digging a hole in the corner of the cell. My fingertips bleed with the effort. I give up.

I have a plan. I will lean on the shower button until I flood the entire courthouse. They'll have to let me out, and I can then slip away unnoticed. In the wardrobe that they provide, this orange jumpsuit ordeal, I hop in the shower and drench myself for maybe an hour. I've never taken a shower for an hour, but I'm doing so now. I'm orange all over, and why orange, I wonder.

The guard tells me to stop. Stop what? I holler. I let up on the shower button, and she asks me if I'm trying to drown myself. My jumpsuit is hot and wet and sticky, and I'm far from amused. However, seeing as how I'm the sharpest knife in the drawer, I tell her yes. Yes, yes, yes, I'm suicidal, I say. I am hoping that maybe they'll take me to a psych unit. There's a bit more room there.

Nope. I ask how many days have gone by. They tell me four or five. How many Law and Order shows am I missing? Am I going to get a lawyer? You did not read me my rights, I scream. So right around then, this other guard unlocks my cell and escorts me down an elevator to another cell where there are a lot of women and a toilet. They aren't lawyers. Everything's orange, everything! Oh my, you'd think I was at a UT bowl game. I can't even pee. I wait and wait and wait. A guard escorts me back to my cell. Somehow, colors are too bright, and what I see are huge distortions. There's a major breakdown in my brain.

The next day, they take me back to that cell downstairs. A social worker comes to see me. I need a lawyer, don't you think? I'm so disappointed. She – the social worker – tells me that she's thinking about letting me see her psychiatrist. You have a psychiatrist? I ask. She says, why yes. So I'm going to go to your appointment instead of you? Why yes, she says again. All she does is confuse me, never gives me an appointment card. Nothing, that's it. At least an appointment card would have been something to hang on to.

I get called to the phone. I'm standing in this little office where the guy hands me the receiver. It's your dad, he says. No lawyer once again. How's your trip going, Dad? I ask. I tell the guy that my dad's on vacation. Do I need to fly up there and help? he asks. No, you don't, but call my doctor. Forget a lawyer.

He says he will, and I know he does. My parents are visiting friends. Dad, enjoy yourself and have a nice day. Just because I'm struggling doesn't mean others can't have a life, I think to myself. That is so very true. I hang up and am escorted back to the cell.

Honestly and not just that it seems so, I'm in jail for over a week, and what was my charge? Yeah, I'd like to know. I'm finally called in front of the judge. I guess that's the closest thing to having a lawyer, I think. By then, I have not slept and have not been on any medication for close to two weeks. When I see the judge, she asks me how I plead. I say Not Guilty. She says, young lady, do you know what perjury is? I say, I know I haven't changed clothes in over a week. Silence, you could hear a pin drop, pardon the cliché, but it's true. Finally catching on, the judge just looks at me, and I see into her warmth. Oh, they screwed up big time, lost in the system, it occurs to me. Maybe because she's perched higher than the rest of us, she can see a bit better.

85

The judge looks really pissed off but not at me. I say I need help, barely able to talk. She says "I know, and I am going to get you that help." Oh no, what am I going to do if she puts me back with that social worker, I think. I say thank you and am escorted back to my cell. I'm bawling my eyes out, thinking I can't take much more. Maybe I'm bawling my eyes out because I'm finally going to get some help.

I stay as glued together as I can, thinking that any minute, I'll feel better. Yet even with the help provided, feeling better is a long way off. Only I don't know it at that moment, and I decide to hang in there. Tell me, what choice do I have? I'm the type of person who is always doing only what I know to do. Don't knock it. Put yourself in my shoes, please, and ask yourself if you really, truly could be doing any better. It's at these times when anything I do perfectly would be considered an accident and maybe even a coincidence. Go team. There's a bigger picture here. Just keep moving the ball down the field, like that judge did that day. I wasn't that far off from helping her. And maybe instead of thinking you could do better or if you criticize me, maybe instead you could simply try to comprehend what all of this feels like.

CHAPTER NINE MORE PSYCHIATRIC UNITS

Well, look at me; you just might be on the wrong floor of this hospital.

It's nighttime. I breathe fresh air, which almost knocks me over. I look down at my feet. Oh, man, I'm still in my orange jumpsuit. Are you taking me home? I ask the police woman who's escorting me out of the jail. Yes, baby, we're taking you home, she says. No, that won't do, I think. Carl is going to kill me, if he's even around.

The cop car pulls up in front of a hospital. So this is my new home, I'm thinking, this isn't good. Nurse Ratched comes to mind; oh no. The cop shows me to a waiting room where there are magazines on a table. One says TIME. Time has stopped, I think. No, times have changed. The past has stopped, and I sit as still as I can in my overwhelming agony. My foot taps the rug with a mind of its own. My shoes smell as bad as the rest of me. I smell like j-a-i-l, like a foul ball.

A guy in regular clothes comes to the door and says it's time to admit me. Can I hang onto this magazine? I ask. Inadvertently, he says sure. He has no clue what I'm going through or what's going to happen next. Oh well, at least I have TIME on my side. Well over a week or more with no sleep, my helpless thoughts do laps around my brain, a mental train wreck, utter distortion. Come on! The guy asks me my name. Fine, I say politely. He writes down Fine where the form says Name. He is sooo nervous. No, fine is how I'm doing. Usually people ask me that first, I say. What's your name? he asks. Well, I'm not fine, I say, far from it. I can't get him to make any sense. We skip to the next section on the form, not doing much better.

He finally asks me my religion; why, I don't know. That's what started this whole mess, I say, an argument about Jesus. Can you believe it? I ask him. The guy seems troubled over no room to write all of that, and I try to help him out: I am lost, put that down. He pauses, seeming to be having a problem finding that on the form. How about 'that far gone' then? Nope. Okay, just put 'other', I say, or 'none'. He sits there. Social worker intern? I ask. He shoots me a look.

Okay, well, Mr. Social Worker intern, I say with perfect enunciation, make a box for me. I point on the form where, and he comes unglued. Where's your supervisor? I ask. She's on vacation, he says. What is it with vacations? Forever vacations. Do people really go there? Yes, he says. Wow, I say in sober disbelief, how cool. Where do people go, their garages?

He says we're done. You know, a box, a square, is it that difficult? I ask. A nurse comes in and asks me if I can muster up some dignity. There I sit, my jumpsuit halfway up my butt, and she raises the issue of dignity? Follow me, she says sternly, which I try to do. I am off balance as I take a deep breath. She shows me my room.

How about 'civilized' for starters, then I'll try for dignity, I think. Maybe she could try a bit, too. I'll try changing. I ask if there are any clothes I can change into. I see clothes on one of the beds in my room. I peel out of my jumpsuit and put on the clothes. My roommate comes in, yelling those are her clothes. Sorry, sorry, sorry, I say quickly. I fly out of them and get back in my jumpsuit. She scares the hell out of me, I tell the nurse, too much commotion for me. I'm holding my head in my hands, trembling. Colors, everywhere.

Jane, we're going to put you in another room, she says. Thank you, I say. The nurse motions for me to follow her. Me? I ask. She nods. Can you speak up, my vision is all over creation,

88

and my ears are stopped up, I say. She sighs heavily and says, this
way, like both syllables are a strain. She shows me a room that has
white walls and a bare mattress on the floor. There is a tiny
window and a slot, like jail. A rubber room? It needs painting,
but that'd heave me even further over the edge.

It's not rubber, I say, as I knock on the walls. My fingers
are still bleeding. This is my room? I ask. For now, she says.
That's TIME terminology, which obviously really messes with
my mind. I say whatever...however...whenever. She leaves me
mumbling, and the door locks with a click.

Another mattress to hug, and I'm still standing, gripping
the hell out of it. I sit down for ten seconds and rise up on tiptoe
for a few moments. I look out the window, and I see many tall
buildings – this must be downtown. There are lights on in some
of the offices. As I look at one building, the lights create a pattern
of words. The words read: Thank you, Jane.

I blink, shake my head and rub my eyes. The words stand:
Thank you, Jane.

Okay, thank me for what? Someone is trying to thank me
in a grandiose fashion in my poor, schizophrenic mind, and I
don't know who to say you're welcome to. You're welcome, I
whisper, and tears run down my cheeks. Reality knocks me to my
knees, and I think, what more can I take? I really am lost and
gone and...what's that word – psychotic.

I have to pee. Oh gosh, I bet it's going to be a damned
ordeal. Some guy comes to the slot and says, "Stand back, and I'll
let you out." I follow him to a bathroom. In mid-trickle that burns
like hell, I get this idea that, if I stand up, I'm going to blow the
whole hospital up with a bomb connected to the toilet. No, that's
just a movie, I try telling myself. Another guy yells, "Stand up
and get back in your room!" I am petrified and begin to cry.
Finally, two guys lift me off the commode in a Queen's chair and

carry me to my door. In utter defeat, I'm covering my ears with my hands, but the kaboom stays crowded in my mind. My head literally hurts. *How is it that I understand them and can talk, somewhat?*

I'm back on my mattress that's covered with a white sheet. Oh no, not the Klan, I'm dead for sure. Where's my doctor? I ask. When will I see the all-too-kind genius who caused this? The Fourth of July is going off in my brain, and I pull on my hair. The voices won't shut up. It just doesn't quit. I have yet to meet anyone who gives a damn. Most of the night, I find myself wishing I'd died in jail. I bet that social worker guy kind of wishes that, too. I really wasn't trying to be all that rude to him. Why do so many therapy people have such trouble with me? I guess I really am that bad. Any vote that it might just be my disorder? And that therapy isn't super effective if you're psychotic?

The next morning, a nurse comes to the slot and says, Jane, we can't have that anymore. What? I ask. She says, your behavior a few hours ago – we can't have that behavior anymore. You can go to the bathroom without the commotion, surely. I tell her with utmost control and composure, Well, look at me, you just might be on the wrong floor of this hospital. I'm gritting really hard, and crack goes another back tooth.

They let me walk around a bit in the day room. The news is on the TV. Did we win the war? I ask. I am so proud to be an American, I shout as I salute. Another nurse says my doctor is here to see me. As usual, he is stern and poised. I'm 'out of it' in most ways possible, which is right up there with 'that far gone', and I ask, Do you know I was in jail for over a week? He looks at the floor. Oh, you bastard, I say, all you had to do was call the courthouse to get me here and back on the right meds. I'm seeing red for the first time in my life. I think: Stop. I take a breath and say to him, *You don't care, do you? You really do not care.* He continues to avoid eye contact.

I march myself back to my 'rubber' room and collapse in my anger, hurt and fear. I cry tears of frustration and sheer loneliness. No one will ever understand what I go through. I talk with my dad who tells me that my doctor refused to take his calls. He says that the doctor knew I was in jail and did nothing. This doctor tries me on Thorazine; I'll never get out.

After a day or two, I feel drugged. I beg the nurses to believe that I'm not using drugs but that I feel drugged. They tell me they know and that they're taking me off it. *Why another antipsychotic?* I ask. *Because there's less of a chance for tardive dyskinesia when you switch antipsychotics,* a nurse tells me. My dad meanwhile feels utterly helpless. I tell him I'm being taken care of, not to worry. Boy, where'd I learn to lie like that?

The doctor gives up and puts me back on my old regimen. After a few days, I get out on a pass. I get to borrow some sweat clothes, which must be Men's Extra Large. I ask a nurse for some tape to use as a belt, which I get all tangled up in my fingers, and I give up. I'll just hang onto the waistband, so I'll need to stay focused. So where might I go? I first call my apartment, and, surprisingly, Carl answers the phone. *Oh, hi,* I say. *Hi,* he says back. *I'm so sorry,* I say. He laughs. *I'm being let out on a pass, and maybe you can come get me,* I suggest, keeping my fingers crossed. *Sure thing,* he says. *I'm glad you called, because I was afraid that they might put you on a medication that would make you not like me,* he confesses. *Oh, save your paranoia, and just come get me,* I say.

My pass is great. A nurse gives me a little plastic plaque that says: PASS. I ask if I can keep it for a souvenir along with my jumpsuit. She laughs and says yes, and I tell her I'm going to put it on my wall in my living room. I do only two things on my

91

pass. I lie on the floor with Carl and watch TV, and I go see a professor at school. The TV is a bit of a problem. I get fed up with our president not wanting to eat his broccoli.

Carl steps out to get stir-fry, and I call The White House, making a huge stink about broccoli. Eat it, you spoiled brat, I say. The guy listens and says he'll relay my concerns. Then it occurs to me I shouldn't have done that. I go sit in the closet where it's quiet and wait for Carl. Would you get a grip? I ask myself.

My pass goes okay when it comes to visiting my professor. He tells me that everyone was trying to get me out of jail. Oh no, that means everyone knows, but what do they know? The professor asks me if my problem is hormonal. I say no, my problem is my doctor. The professor looks at me, trying not to laugh. It cues me in. I add that my problem is chemical, neuro-hormonal. I say, I guess I need to pack up my things. You are moving? he asks. Um, not right away, I'm quitting school, I say. He asks, Why? I say, Well, surely you don't want me here. I had prepared myself for the news, but not the news I got.

Jane, you are a good student, we aren't wishing you'd leave. Sometimes people get sick, he says. So what can we do to help you? he asks. I want to postpone my internship, I say. He says they can arrange that. He'd like me to meet with the faculty when I feel up to it.

I see a phone and call Dr. Jobson. What is it with your referrals? I say. I explain, and he says that doctor was the best. I say, gritting my teeth again and again, Dr. Jobson, the fact that someone has the most expensive office furniture does not make him the best doctor. Why am I so compelled to state the obvious for people? See you later, I say, and I hang up.

I walk around campus and glance at a school newspaper. This is the year my back teeth are ground down to nothing. There's a research associate position coming available in a few weeks. I ask my adviser about it. He makes some phone calls and finds out that I would need to defend my dissertation to be eligible. Some doors are still open to me. I focus on that.

I go back to the hospital. A normal mattress awaits my hug. Man, the things that become my comfort zones, like mattresses, closets, driving...they become quite the habits to break. I vow never to go back to that psychiatrist. I'm not the only one trying to protect me, but it sure feels that way sometimes. I call my parents and tell them all about it. I tell them sorry for somewhat ruining their vacation, if I did. I never do these things on purpose. Goodness, you'd think people would know that. My parents don't know what to think except they say they're sorry for what I go through. At least someone is tuned in.

I tell them that Carl has been great; he's a musician, played guitar on the Opry for 16 years, and he really cares. They tell me they're glad I have him, and that's probably going to be the only time they say that. I tell them I'm going to try to find my part-of-a-dissertation draft on my computer. They say, Oh my, we hope you find it. We love you. Keep us posted.

Some people might think that my parents should cut me out of the family or drop me off at a shelter. Some people might think that they should have stormed the jail and busted me out, all while having a heart attack. Me, though, honestly? I think my parents were perfect for staying in Florida and using the phone. If I had needed them in person, and they were willing (which they were), I would have screamed 911 all over everywhere. And guess what? My parents would have died trying to help me. It's a problem for me, having to protect them from my problems. I would have 'died' over my dad racing to my side and having a heart attack. He'd do that.

My disorder is painful in jail, every kind of pain. Yet it's when I am out and about that I could get killed. All I'm saying is *that it's dangerous for me when I'm disordered. There are many unexpected ways to die even with a perfect safety plan in place. Think about the vulnerabilities...stepping in front of a car, meeting up with the wrong people, being robbed at knife point, being in a rough neighborhood...*

Three weeks later and back on my old medication, I'm allowed to go. With no time to think, I meet with the clinical director and my favorite professor, not the entire faculty. Either way, I feel supported by them. They never ask my diagnosis, and I give them Dr. Jobson's phone number so that they can call and ask away. They never do. Why would they trust me? Because they know me?

I get busy on my dissertation, because I need that research job. I'm about down to pennies, and Carl is trying to find work. It takes what seems like years to get reacquainted with the partial draft of my dissertation. I finally do. My topic has to do with helping friends in need, helping one another when it comes to health problems. I realize that I lost almost my entire support system over a medication alteration. Some support system, I think to myself. When I really need people, they are often nowhere to be found. In my dissertation, I find that only when people are really bored do they help others. I wonder if 'bored' goes a bit deeper, but that was the word indicated. Maybe it has to do with time and kindness. I don't know. Is it really such a thing as, I don't have anything to do, I think I'll help a friend?

I do believe that it is difficult to help anyone who is psychotic and, in a different way, difficult to help anyone who is dying. I also realize that people are often truly busy. There are people, however, who truly care and who make the time to help, and my hat is off to these people. Sure, we need to take care of ourselves, but I'm talking about just moments of caring. A kind gesture often takes just a moment and can make a world of

94

difference.

***

Carl and I are in the living room. We talk about what to do with ourselves. He laughs about some of the things I say and do when I'm disordered. We have some private laughs. Our charges are dropped. What was I arrested for, Carl, do you know? I ask. Being yourself, he says. Thanks, you jerk. He says, you had me arrested. I say, I know, sorry, but you got out that night, how'd that happen? He just looks at me and smiles. Did I tell you I called The White House and told them to tell George to shut up and eat his broccoli? Carl says, No way, Jane. Seriously, I say.

A few hours go by. Carl is trying to vacuum without sucking up the cord, and I am trying to put pages of my dissertation in numerical order. Only I didn't number the pages, what a mess. It doesn't occur to me to get on the word program, number the pages and print it. No, that'd make too much sense. Actually, I am out of ink cartridges and can't buy another one until I get my paycheck next week.

The phone rings. Carl hops up to answer. Hello? He looks at me and says, I think it's for you. Who is it? I ask. He says, It's The White House. See, Carl, I told you I called them, I holler, jumping up and down. Jane, stop jumping up and down, it makes me nervous. He shoves the phone toward me, his arm outstretched. Take the phone, Jane. Take the damn phone. Take the bleeping phone. You don't have to say it like that, I say, grabbing the receiver. Mr. Jesus and all – you shouldn't swear, Carl.

Hello? I say. Oh, hi. I'm fine; well, I'm better. I'm back on the right medication. I appreciate you checking up on me. That's very nice. Tell our president that there are a lot of people who have problems that he'll never understand, and you have a nice day. You give me hope, I add, hanging up the phone. Who was it?

95

Carl asks. Some lady, I say. Maybe the president's mother, I don't know. No, a clerk or someone. I think they screen calls and check up on crazy people, like, do they need help. That's amazing.

Not a dull moment with you, Carl says.

I'm sorry about the trouble I've caused; I didn't do anything on purpose, I say quietly. He puts his arms around me and says, I know, baby, I know. Then he starts laughing.

Is everything just a big joke for you? I ask. No, but come on, Jane, come on. Where we going? I ask. Wherever we're going, we're going together, he says. I smile about that.

CHAPTER TEN BECOMING A DOCTOR

...can you tell when I'm disordered, and am I funny?

August 28, 2009

Maybe Jane will show up. I have no control over what my clients say and do. Especially Jane. It's like trying to pick up mercury. I do realize that her unique talents are truly beyond anything I've accomplished. Some people are unusual and phenomenal, and I've decided to sit back and watch.

I vow to say things that can be as helpful and supportive as possible, like 'good job', 'high five' and maybe even 'way to go'. She always laughs when I say such things, and I love to hear her laugh. She says I'm a nerd. I say thanks. The truth is that many people are blessed, and very few are chosen. Jane's chosen. She has trouble seeing it, though. However, I do think we're getting somewhere.

Jane shows for her appointment today. She asks me how I'm doing. Good, I say. I tell her that she's been through a lot. She readily agrees. Carolyn, she asks, am I funny? I mean, can you tell when I'm disordered, and am I funny? I smile. Play the right card, I say to myself. I think so, I say. I think so.

So you can tell, and I'm funny?

"Yes and yes, but Jane, you..." Jane smiles and cuts in.

I don't mean to be funny. Sometimes, though, I laugh at situations. I do break through quite a few myths. Everyone who has a "chemical imbalance" has his or her own personality. Maybe it's kind of funny when a certain part of my disorder is showing through my personality. It can be, at times, funny, later.

I'm so kind and serious that people think I'm being a jerk. Carolyn, what do you think?

Hmm. I notice that she's calling me Carolyn, but I don't tell her that I notice.

"Well, you're not a jerk. I do believe you were an outstanding graduate student. And I believe that you struggle with a "chemical imbalance" that's highly demanding and serious in nature. I'm so sorry, and yet it's amazing. I also think that you're a very kind, very intelligent person who needs to take good care. And you definitely go the extra mile for yourself and others." Jane seems to ignore me.

Well, some aspects of graduate school were a breeze. Actually, all of it was easy until my adviser and best friend died. I seriously grieved, because I was so close to them. I really missed them.

My disorder has been way more than a full-time job, and boy, do I have to be intelligent to live my life, or what? It's taken me 33 years to be who I am today, and I'm still on the mend from what happened a couple of years ago. It's tiring and discouraging to have to start over and over, especially when it's not something I've done. It's doctors, med changes, dosage changes, side effects...I guess I can explain that later. Do you want to hear how I met Carl?

"Sure."

I'll be in touch.

Clear the way, leaving her appointment early, there she goes. Damn! I'm starting to feel as if her therapy isn't working for me. I call a colleague who tells me to roll with it, that something's working for *Jane.*

She writes:

It's my fourth year of graduate school, and I haven't dated

98

the whole time. I'm getting ready to turn 30 years old. Oh, man, it's not right, turning 30 and still a virgin. I think that could very well be a sin or maybe just blasphemous. I've got to do something, I'm thinking. I was born at 3:00 a.m., and I need to hurry. I call a friend and tell him my problem. He says he'll be right over, and he shows up in ten seconds. Later I tell him that sex is over-rated. He says thanks. I say you're welcome.

A couple of days later, I'm standing on the front porch of the house where my efficiency is. This guy in blue jeans and cowboy boots walks by. He's tall and slim, some graying hair. He walks down the alley to the back. I don't think much about it except, This guy is cute.

So the guy downstairs calls me. He asks me if I want to come down and eat fish. I say sure. So I meet Carl, the guy I saw in the alley a moment ago, and he is staying on this other guy's couch. Well, the guy starts to get pissed about Carl and me talking and laughing. So this guy pulls out a gun. Why'd I pick a place to live one block from campus?

I grab Carl's shirt and tug. We go racing out the door and to my apartment. I'm huffing and puffing, and I say, Carl, we need to move. So we wait until the next day, and we find an apartment and shove all of my stuff in my car. Carl's stuff is still in his car, but he can't get his car started. He grabs his clothes and, his car? He says to forget about it, that he only paid $200 for it. So we move, and that's that.

Here I am, living with a guy I just met. That was never how I planned things. Carl, however, is an amazing performer, and I go to where he gets a job and watch him wow crowds. He's really good. He's performed all over the world. We really hit it off. He's on a comeback from having his hand cut badly when he fell on a broken beer bottle left behind by who knows who, while he was fishing. He and I have an understanding. We're both very *talented and have experienced bad luck and need each other.*

After a week or so, I go see that psychiatrist, and you know what happens then. Carl hangs in there with me, and how can I not like him? He's a great guy, very caring and loving. Why couldn't I have waited a couple of days on the sex thing? I can be so impatient, if 29-year old virgins can even be that.

***

I prepare myself for defending my dissertation. Then, I am surrounded by five men, all of whom are the best in their areas of study. I think it was harder to get them all in the same place at the same time than it was doing my dissertation, but I managed. They ask me to explain what I have learned from doing my dissertation. I discuss my findings and offer interpretations.

I think they probably know a little about me and being in jail and the hospital. I continue to answer their academic questions, which was tough, and then I'm asked what I would say if I were eating dinner with my family. I say, well, a lot of people are too busy to help, but there are some chosen few who are very kind and who care for the sake of being kind. Still, they need to have boundaries, set limits. Silence.

I wonder if she is actually going to become a doctor at this point. I'm amazed that she's just out of jail, having been lost in the system for over a week and then three weeks in the hospital and trying to complete this milestone at this time, one week later. I smile at her audacity and fearlessness. I want to tell her she's got guts. I have an inkling that I would have quit school, but not Jane. And she wanted the research job *bad*. She loves research. She's not easily deterred, just putting one foot in front of the other.

Jane continues:

Well, I don't set things up. All I know to do is try to be a good person. I try not to think about the people who scatter when

I get sick, although I get very sad at times. I guess I have who I need. My dissertation committee members are very hard on me but fair. They think I'm tuned in, which I am.

I'm asked to step out of the room for them to deliberate. I step into the women's restroom and look in the mirror. I think back to age 20, touching the glass...what I've been through...I tell myself that it's going to be okay, no matter what. I know I could fail. I know that explaining myself didn't go so well, because explaining anything has been hard for me to do since I first got sick at age 16. I touch the glass and tell myself I'm here. You're trying, I say, and that counts for something.

My chairperson comes out of the room. I hear the door squeak as it opens, and he calls my name. I walk back in the room and sit quietly at the table, all eyes on me. This is it. They are all so serious. Oh my.

It's unanimous, Jane.

I ask, what is? They all smile. You passed, he says. I shake their hands, say thanks and run the mile home. I jump into Carl's arms, having known him for just a couple of months but feeling as if I've known him for a lifetime. He gives me a big hug.

I need to call my parents. There is no answer, but they know I was defending my dissertation. The phone rings. It's my parents, who stop driving long enough to tell me they're just half an hour away. They tell me they're coming over to celebrate. What if I hadn't passed? I ask my dad. He says, then we'd be there to be supportive and to talk about what you could do with your life. Well, we've had that discussion many a time, but not this day.

That reminds me, I need to call about the research job, I say. I hang up and call the professor who posted the job notice. He gives me the job over the phone. I smile and breathe. So is this what a life can be? Wow! Things go easy for me for a couple of

101

weeks, which feels almost too unusual, as I polish my dissertation.

***

Every time a doctor changes meds on me, I have to start over. I've changed careers or have started over, let's see, how many times? I don't even want to count. I get moved back to Go, don't collect $200, while everyone is racing around the board, buying property and having a good ole' time. I've also spent a lot of time in jail, rolling three times before getting out. You know how to play Monopoly, don't you, Carolyn?

You'll see that I actually end up working as a tech at a treatment center twice. *And my résumé is not that bad. I have done some good work. It's enough for people to think I've done well as a doctor. If they only knew! I'm not complaining, Carolyn. I'm hoping that my illness is treated well enough and allows me to be the full me some day. Plus I'm always wishing for a friend or two who understands!*

Maybe, if I'm ever ready, the things that have gone wrong in my life will someday be beautiful. I think it's somewhere in Africa, some tribe where members who are delusional are considered godlike. I'd be right up there, wouldn't I? Seriously, though, beautiful would be if I have helped even just one person with my story. If my pain and humiliation could help someone, that would be beautiful. Or if what I do that works could help a lot of people.

***

August 26, 2009

Why am I not surprised that Jane drops off an abundance of reading but doesn't stay? I place the pages in my purse and start my workday. My life mostly goes unnoticed, and I like that. It gives me some privacy and allows me to have a decent relationship with myself. My mother says she made mistakes with me. Thanks, I tell her.

102

Then, following my sarcasm, I ask what she means by that. Well, you stay so much to yourself, she says. And? I say. No, that's all, she says.

It kind of pisses me off, but she's my mother. What would she have done differently with me? . My mother, the psychologist, who does she think she is, making a mistake with me? Well, I like me, I mumble, as I pull out of my parent's driveway, and you didn't have to have me, I whisper. I know she loves me.

I wonder about Jane's parents. She told me, one session, that she has often been very angry with her parents for having her. Yet she has a sister who is a world-famous scientist and who also has a wonderful husband and two great kids. There's nothing 'wrong' with *her*. She has a huge home, travels the world and is very happy.

One time, Jane told me that a family friend said, "How can someone as nice as Jane have so many problems?" This family friend also called Jane and told her that it was time for her to buy a house. Buy a house between medication changes? The problem that would cause! Kids, houses, vacations, awards, celebrations...these things didn't get put in her schedule. Jane told me that these things were just not realistic, not reality-based in her journey. It doesn't bother her that much unless someone points it out with a shaming finger. Jane knows how very much her disorder has held her back.

That's something I try to provide for Jane, an understanding and a desire to comprehend what she has done and had to do. I get a glimpse of her genius. She doesn't see it, busy trying to be 'normal' or who others think she should be. She gets caught up in the spokes of a wheel defined by others. When will she learn that's not the way to go, not the place to ride? When will she let go of some image she tries to live up to? What's the point of trying to appear normal? Why not be herself?

Jane tells me that there are a lot of things I just don't get. Me, normal? That'd be nice. I say, fair enough, and keep listening. My God, it occurs to me that she's riding a bike while trying to fix it...along with trying to help others fix...and she's *doing* it. She cares a lot.

Jane says that she learns something every day about her illness. That's 33 years x 365 days. She breaks it down to an art of developing an awareness and being able to communicate that awareness. I finally ask her the name of her illness. Jane says that, after she defended her dissertation, she visited Dr. Jobson and asked him. He first asked her what *she* thought. She said that she thought it was a very biologically-based, major mental illness.

From the drugs I'm on and knowing my symptoms, she said, *I'd say manic-depressive illness and schizophrenia, all rolled up in one.* She then said, *Dr. Jobson, it's a chronic, very severe schizo-affective disorder.* Dr. Jobson said yes, and that he'd never seen a more severe case and one that responded well to medication. It definitely helps.

The medication takes care of a lot but also gets me in touch enough for me to struggle with the rest, Jane says. Dr. Jobson may or may not fully comprehend what Jane does to stay centered. There are so many things she does that help once medication gives her a leg up. Jane's not even sure what she does that works for her, how to explain it in some organized fashion.

Jane tells me that she thinks it was some type of schizophrenia all along. She says it unnerved her for her parents to say she was bipolar and easily treated. Is that why it took six years to diagnose her and find the right medications? They don't want to see her struggle. And so Jane walks that line, really struggling but trying not to inconvenience or worry others.

Jane told me, one session, that she experienced a dose of harsh reality when she saw patients in the state mental hospital. These were the most chronic, severely mentally ill patients an intern would ever see. Jane was assigned to a young woman who had schizo-affective disorder. This woman was even on the same medications as Jane. When Jane met this patient, she was whisked into a world of King Arthur's court. Every now and then, there was a window where this patient's true and current life shone through. Jane tried to encourage that.

One day, this patient was riding on a stationary bicycle, and Jane asked her what was it about our world, why not live out and about, maybe at home with her parents? She got really mad at Jane and said, "It's obvious." Jane knew that this patient became sick when she was 20 years old and a student at a top university.

What's obvious?

"People don't like people like me. People here are nice to me." That was the end of it. The patient refused to ever talk with Jane again. I asked Jane how she felt about that experience.

Sad and angry and scared. Sad for her. Angry with society. And scared for me. I walked away, because it was time. And because I didn't want to know just precisely what it was that people did to her. Once again, what's so difficult about being nice?

CHAPTER ELEVEN DRINKING BEER

...my second problem started out being a solution.

Dr. Dobbins,

I've put the following behind me:

I spent a year in the research position, working only 40 hours per week, and it gave me enough free time with Carl for me to know how much I loved him. I only had two problems that year. One was that I was on a very low dosage of my medications. As always, my sleep was fitful, and I was constantly afraid of waking up psychotic. I ended up in jail two more times. Same drill, but not as many days behind bars. It wore me out. More people found out, and I started feeling as if I didn't deserve being on campus. It was such a frightening and angering existence that I stopped caring much about myself but still wanted a solution any which way I could get it.

My second problem started out being a solution. With what friends I had left and more time on my hands, I started going to Happy Hour. I soon found out that beer knocked me out and allowed me to sleep. The only problem was, I had to drink more and more for the same effect. I found myself always with a beer in my hand, which kept me sedated. It kept me from getting psychotic, but it took away at least half of my intelligence.

Carl became concerned. My parents knew I was drinking. I didn't care that alcohol was smearing my shine. I couldn't see any existence worth living – thanks a lot, too-much-beer. All I had was one year of clinical work and an exam to become a licensed psychologist, but I lost sight of the light at the end of the tunnel. I woke up with the shakes. I knew nothing about chemical dependence or treatment. I learned nothing about all of that in graduate school. Two years went by. What did I do?

My parents were angry and told me not to visit them unless I got help. Carl said he'd leave me, too, if I didn't get help. Upon completion of the research job, I went to treatment at a four-month program and stayed seven months. They started me out in detox and then dropped me with a thud in the psych unit. My roommate jumped in the swimming pool with a big "Yippee" and a huge splash and all her clothes on. She got strapped down, and so I made a point of sitting as still as possible.

Eventually, I was dropped off at an apartment complex. I had graduated to residential treatment, and I slung my bags on what some woman told me was my bed. She then drove me to a building where there were people everywhere. I blended in as quietly as possible. I followed the crowd outside, where most of them smoked, and then to a lecture hall where a guy showed slides and then into a car and back to the apartment. My bags were not on my bed.

I looked everywhere. They were in the living room. I put them back in my room and introduced myself to my roommate. She neither looked up nor said anything. The other two women in the apartment were equally friendly. I went outside for some air and started crying. I wiped away my tears and tried again. My bags were on the patio. I went back outside until dark and came back in. The three of them were in their rooms, and I dragged my bags in from the patio and sat on the couch until morning.

I guess word got around that I came from the psych unit. I met my counselor and told her what happened. She told me I had to confront my fellow travelers in group. I dodged a panic attack, simply breathing heavily and looking at the carpet. I was afraid of everything. I'm not sure what I said, but some of them seemed to side with me. I earned a bed to sleep in, although my roommate still wouldn't talk to me. I decided I didn't care.

I did my homework assignments on a typewriter because

my hands shook all of the time. The psychiatrist, who was young and arrogant, told me that I wasn't weird enough to be schizo-affective. I asked him to call Dr. Jobson, which he didn't do. I also reminded him that I was medicated. He still wanted me off the antipsychotic medication. Here we go again. I was scared to death of freaking out in my apartment.

Three times, the psychiatrist lowered my meds, and each time, I caught some early symptoms without there being an upset, mainly just low grade hallucinations. Nonetheless, he said that he was diagnosing me as bipolar -- pretty much to give me a crack at treatment, as the staff felt someone who was schizo-affective could not make it through the program. Well, aside from tampering with my diagnosis, what are you going to do with me, I asked. If I were you, I said, I'd keep me on the meds I got here on and up them instead of lower them. He did. Don't ask me what they said about me in staffings, but I did well during my over-extended stay.

After four months, the staff spent three months looking for a group home for me, couldn't find one that would take someone with my (severe) diagnosis and just let me go. Out the door. It was an experience opposite to what I would call faith-building. It was as if they were afraid of, not so much me, but my diagnosis. I would never have been able to tolerate the way I was treated by most of the clients had it not been for my counselor. She was open to having me try for a life, and she was just plain respectful and encouraging.

***

One morning, I woke up with a really bad cough and felt drained. I asked to see the physician. He told me to get some rest. I wasn't getting any better. I went back. Same answer. Then one night, I got up to get some orange juice, and I fell and couldn't get up. I hollered for help, and no one came to help me. I finally

108

made it back to bed.

The next morning, I went to my counselor. She had me taken to the ER. The doctor said I had double or triple pneumonia, whichever, and I literally almost died. The physicians were very worried about me and kept me in the hospital for over a week. They were furious over what had happened to me and kept a very close eye on me.

Treatment was the worst experience ever in many ways, but I stayed there in order to have a successful discharge. I was making sure that I never had to go back. No one on the staff thought I'd ever be able to stay sober. It was as if my mental disorder did not give me the control I needed not to drink. For me, the issue was more that I could abstain from drinking if I were ever allowed enough of the antipsychotic drug. I understand wanting the lowest dosage possible to ward off debilitating side effects, but...I tried to be patient and see the good in being there.

I learned about the 12 steps. I went to meetings and groups. Honestly, I felt depressed and exhausted. Carl was a great support to me and visited whenever he could. He got involved in my treatment and wanted the best for me and for us. I never wanted to say goodbye to him. He cared, and he thought that I could do whatever I set my mind to doing. I loved him more than anyone.

I was finally discharged and went back to living with Carl in our apartment in Nashville. He and I both wanted to move. I felt that I'd never have much of a chance building a practice there. And honestly, I didn't want to be a psychologist at all. I was exhausted from everything that had happened to me, especially the negativity about my prognosis expressed to me in treatment. The dread of living with my disorder for a lifetime, or even from one day to the next, overwhelmed me. I saw myself never working again or doing anything else. Any effort seemed pointless, life, *just a chore. And much of this, it seemed, was coming from the staff and clients. I internalized it, because I really did feel that unwanted, that put down. I mean, they cared; they just didn't have much hope for me. They imposed limits on me that they had learned from...where? A stereotype? A diagnostic manual? Other patients with my disorder?*

Carl had this idea that we could move to Florida and perform together. I haven't told you this, but I learned to play the guitar as a teenager. I also sang for fun, and he wanted me to sing with him. I was against the idea because Carl was really good. I was not. Oh, I could carry a tune, but I never thought of myself as a performer. Anyway, he bought this band machine and started programming all these great songs that I loved – traditional country, 60s music...And he made me sing with him. I started having fun, tried to focus on great things that were fun.

We loaded up, moved to Florida, and played up and down the coast. We bought a little trailer to live in, and I was really happy in our little group home of Carl and me. Wherever we performed, mainly in restaurants, people said "You guys need to go to Branson!" So we did. In two years, we were doing shows in various theaters and having a great time. We could have made more money, if Carl had put a little more into it, as he did with fishing. He cared nothing about money and couldn't see that it was hurting us, but it was. I told him that I'd get a job – any job. I had medical and dental bills to pay.

I landed a job selling timeshares and got fired for not measuring up, not making enough sales. I guess I was too busy listening to people's problems. I did go to AA meetings and stayed sober, though, for two years. I stayed on my medication and yet never really slept well, no matter the dosage. Sometimes symptoms kept me awake, and insomnia could also produce symptoms. The main concern was that I wasn't psychotic.

110

So there in the midst of my life, I picked up a newspaper. There was a part-time job advertised for a tech at an Alcohol and Drug treatment center. I got excited and nervous over that ad, all at once. Could I even manage? I decided to give it a try.

Before I started work, Carl and I decided we'd get married. Planning it was really stressful, and I found myself really worried that "stress" would send me over the edge. My parents didn't seem to understand what I loved about Carl. He cared about me, that I know. No, he adored me and loved me completely. The ceremony itself was beautiful, and I don't quite know how I pulled it off. I bought my wedding dress at a thrift store for one dollar, but I felt as if it was worth a million bucks. It was beautiful.

Everyone seemed to have a good time, especially Carl and me. We just ignored things about our families who created more tension than necessary. I guess it was always expected of me to marry someone who was wealthy, and that just didn't happen. After so many years of living with Carl, it seemed right to have the wedding – and I managed to stay well through the whole ordeal.

We then went about our business. I still sang with Carl, and I got the job at the center. I bought a Chevrolet Celebrity for $400, and you'd think I landed a brand new Mercedes. Only it didn't have any brakes. I found that out the hard way, and I'm not even going to explain the full version – I closed my eyes, said oh shit or oh no or both and coasted to a stop with the help of a curb that kept me from gliding into the front window of a store.

The job at the center went okay. I didn't tell anyone I had a PhD, for fear they'd ask questions I wouldn't know how to answer, such as, "What are you doing here? Shouldn't you be a professor at some big university?" I had lost touch with my *soaring reputation in graduate school. My disorder, alcohol and treatment had reduced me down to size, and I was only interested in being the me I could be at the center. That's all I had. I set my sights on staying employed.*

My shift was 3-11 p.m. Looking back, I can see that my biggest problem was that I had started to believe the professionals who told me I couldn't do anything professionally, a career. In a way, they were right. Maybe I should even say that I shouldn't have been able to hold down any job, forget career. At work, I had trouble explaining things. My thoughts were scattered. Things that were sitting there moved, and I tried not to jump. I tried to focus on work tasks. Looking back, I think my symptoms were exacerbated for a period of time, as I was getting used to a new job, new surroundings.

And so I took detox clients' blood pressures. I handed residential clients toiletries from the closet. I was so proud of myself for handing clients the right items. I answered the phones. When they were all in bed by 10:30, I did cartwheels down the hallways. I built my confidence up rather quickly. Whatever I needed to do, from moment to moment, I could do. Of course, I thought too much. And I stayed internally upset over how I was doing, but I didn't get fired after any shift. I kept on showing up. I kept being told, "Oh, you're doing such a great job..."

One night, though, I had a close call. I wore a white lab coat with big pockets in which I carried the portable phone. I had to pee and needed to make it to the bathroom fast. When I stood up, the phone slid into the toilet. I left a note for all the staff to see; something like: Sorry, do I still have a job? I'll pay for it...and everyone thought I had this amazing sense of humor, while I was serious! One of the other techs blew the phone dry with a hair dryer, and that was it, dial tone again. Onto the next crisis.

Well, the next problem I had was a bit different. The

director came to the tech station and told me that there was no one to teach anger management, so I would be doing that. Ordinarily, only counselors and senior techs were allowed to teach a class, but I would have to do. I rarely talked, so how was this going to work? No time for minor technicalities. The director shoved the lecture material my way with no chance for me to protest. I could feel panic coming on.

I walked into the classroom and went to the front, leaning on a podium. I said hi, my name is Jane. They said, We know. Then something hit me on my forehead, and then again and again. And sitting on the podium were spitballs. That's cute, you guys, I said. Whoever did this, pick these up after class, please. I looked at the lecture and realized I had no clue what the words said, not a clue. What then?

This was one of my first attempts after treatment to allow my mouth to open without practicing what I would say in my mind first. I think I said, Okay, this is anger management. Then I stopped. Whiz came another spitball, missing me by a yard. Bad aim, I said, and left it at that. Here I go again with opening my mouth. Anyone mad about anything? Silence. No spit balls. No one? Anyone mad about being an alcoholic or addict? I asked. No one said a word.

Okay, I said, I'd say I'm angry at times about being an alcoholic. Something as seemingly trivial as a foamy, gold-colored liquid reduced me to my knees, and I couldn't get up. I went to treatment, and admittedly, I hated it. However, I'm alive today and am two years sober. And maybe by being here, I can help a fellow alcoholic or addict.

Then with what had to be nothing short of a miracle, they started chiming in and discussing how they got where they were that day. We started conversing, and my anxiety subsided. The director walked in and said she liked what she was hearing. Did she know that I had ditched the lecture? I don't know. I think I just got lucky. When class finished, I stood at the podium, waiting to see if anyone was going to throw away the spitballs. A woman who looked to be in her 60s came up to the podium, picked up the spitballs and said, Sorry. I about died laughing, thinking it had been the younger guys who were guilty. You never know about people.

I managed to keep my job and relax a bit. An older male counselor cornered me in the tech station one day and asked me how I knew so much. What do you mean? I asked. He said that I used the terminology of someone schooled in psychology and counseling. Okay, I said...and I told him my background and swore him to secrecy. That turned out well.

The next morning I was in the director's office, when she asked me to work as a counselor. I said I'd give it a try. So a counselor I became, nervous and afraid of everything and then some. I figured that if it was supposed to be this way, I'd go with it, which I did with flying colors.

Amazingly, a couple of years went by. I became clinical director for a few years and then the director for six years. I loved my job, staying there eleven years. I worked very hard, 50-70 hours per week, and became interested in doing everything I could to help the clients and staff at the center. I networked and reached out to and connected with mental health providers, mainly psych units, but also churches, halfway houses and domestic violence shelters. I tagged any affiliation that could help clients who had substance abuse problems as well as mental illnesses. Once again, I started with the Yellow Pages. There were quite a few clients who had bipolar disorder or schizophrenia. They left treatment lined up with jobs instead of disability. Many of them stayed sober and experienced an increased quality of life.

Methamphetamine was a huge problem in this area of

Missouri, and law enforcement was always ready to show. One guy put his arm through a glass window pane, and the sheriff took him to the hospital to be stitched up and given some medication to calm him down. I learned how to side-step and duck quite readily. Most of the clients were poor, and although I understand needing money, meth labs and sales are clearly illegal. Some clients went to prison and came back on probation. My passion was stupendous, and I simply remember one counselor who said, "Jane's clients stay sober." Hmm, pretty much.

I became very well known in the area. The staff and I made connections with probation offices and set up education programs for Drug Court. For those eleven years, I adjusted to my symptoms, which were minimal, and then I almost forgot about the severity I had endured. People said I was a legend. That flipped me out. I was just busy in the trenches, serving a population in great need. I was honored to function and honored to serve. It was a rough job, to say the least, but I was exceedingly happy and challenged. I felt a joy and freedom that I had only dreamed of.

I loved those people -the staff, the clients and any contacts outside of the center. We were quite the collective miracle. Being there those eleven years was the highlight of my professional life. I think I did well, because the set-up allowed me to take care of the center, through having the freedom to take care of my disorder, i.e., set my own schedule and calling the shots. I also think that, when I work hard, I sleep better.

CHAPTER TWELVE A MIRACLE

Oh, who knows why I do the things the way I do?

Jane has an energy that she puts to good use. Her passion is helping others. Her life has been scattered to pieces, and she works hard to pick them up and try again. It's hard for her to see how unusual she is, how amazing she is. I see it, and I don't know if she ever will. She seems too busy being caught up in humility, being teachable. Even in the face of moderate symptoms, she knowingly tries to approach normal every moment.

My receptionist calls. Jane is here. Oh, good, I think. I have a lot of questions for her, if she's willing to respond. She says hi as she walks in. She sits down and smiles. So where are we at? I ask. I'm not sure, she says. Well, why did you write that last set in past tense and not as if you were living it? I ask.

I'm not sure. Maybe because it's easier to admit to and accept my life in that last set of pages. It's as if I were able to admit all of what I wrote did happen – my alcohol problem came and went, my disorder never goes away. It's always in the present. An alcohol problem is different than my disorder. It seems to be more easily to overcome, for me, anyway.

"What are you saying, that you're not an alcoholic? Or you are?"

Well, I think I was self-medicating so I could sleep and wouldn't get psychotic. I abused alcohol and became dependent on it. When I'm on the right medication and am stable, alcohol doesn't mean anything to me. I don't like it or crave it when I'm properly medicated. Alcoholic or not, I went to AA meetings and grew to love alcoholics and addicts.

"And when you're off your meds?"

When I'm off my meds or the dosage is too low, I have little control over anything. That would include drinking, and my brain knows alcohol keeps me sedated. So I use it. However, after treatment, I stayed sober for 13 years and certainly sober while working at the center, out of respect for the clients and scared of alcohol, even when I wasn't sleeping well. I guess I'll never really sleep well. As long as I don't get psychotic, I don't complain.

"So you went from a part-time tech, worrying about keeping your job, to the director, in how many years, at a 32-bed facility?" I can't help but laugh over such irony.

Maybe five years, three or so of those years as clinical director. We also had a huge outpatient program. I think it was all supposed to happen that way. Every day, things could have played out any which way. I felt so blessed to be able to roll up my sleeves and be a productive member of society. So many people complain about their jobs or having to work. That's insane to me.

Every day, I could go home and say, I made it through another day. What a blessing. Don't get me wrong, it was tough. Man, that job was tough, no way a full career job. Everyone in the director job seemed to fizzle after about 3-5 years. Those eleven years were hard. *But I had the freedom to create, and no one micromanaged me. All I heard was sort of like, go girl, from my boss! I was very trustworthy, could think on my feet and also be thoughtful. I really, really cared.*

"Like that surprises me, Jane."

Oh, sorry.

"No need to be. What did you do about becoming a psychologist?"

Well, I'm a PhD psychologist, but not licensed as one. When I saw that I could work full-time as a counselor/director,

117

and with all that I did – the good that happened – I opted to go a different route and not quit for a year just to complete an internship at a designated site for licensure as a psychologist. A friend of mine suggested I look into becoming licensed as a counselor. It would at least allow me to stay in my job, and it would allow me to have some freedom in seeing clients with mental health problems. At that time, I was certified as a substance abuse counselor. So I looked into the suggestion.

I had to be supervised for a year, and it was worth it. I mean, my supervisor was outstanding. First, I had to go to night school and take several counseling classes at a nearby university. You'd think all the classes I took to get a doctorate would do, but the counseling board said it had to be counseling classes! Long story short, I got a license in counseling. This was good, because I had always wanted to go into private practice at some point.

"You really know how to adjust."

No, it was that those clients and the staff at the center meant the world to me. I've always more or less looked for opportunities to have a life, to fill a need. I've also very often felt like quite the failure. Imagine being in medical school and then years later, I'm a tech at a treatment center. But let me say this: I loved being a tech. I was so effective in that job, because clients tell techs things they don't tell the rest of the staff. And it's hard to be a good tech. You really have to be on your toes. And it really helped me get on my feet. I enjoyed that job.

I still valued being the director, actually the associate director. (There was no director.) I worked very hard and had a lot of good leadership qualities..I usually find something to help me make sense of it all. For example, what am I doing here in Branson and also the middle of meth capitol USA, singing and running a treatment center? Trying to do good and help out, that's all. That's just where I got put.

118

Well, for as long as I can remember, I've thought that there's something much bigger and better than I – a power, all good. I'm just me, and I just try to do the right things. I've always been that way, and a good sport when you look at my life, always happy for others, always wanting to help if someone needs some support, sometimes tough on the staff and clients. Not much good has come of my life in terms of rewards, and my life has been a really rough go, for certain. However, with work, the reward should be the work itself, you know? Believe me, I enjoyed myself.

"I see."

Anyway, life with Carl was going okay. I still sang with him some; the crowds were huge. I typically watched him perform quite a bit. It was tough to both work and sing. We started making really good money as time went on.

I kept growing spiritually in Branson. I learned things like 'everything happens for a reason' and 'things work out the way they're supposed to'. I received a chemistry from who-knows-where, but that doesn't make me a bad person by any means. And honestly, I'm not sure what spirituality is. I guess it's about choices, the choices we make and why. I think spirituality has to do with certainty in a higher power and in caring.

"Do you feel remarkable?"

Sometimes I do, and then sometimes I don't. Sometimes I'm amazed. Other times, I'm just a burden to myself.

"You've done a lot of footwork."

I won't argue with you on that. I just don't see what good it has done. You know, diabetics used to be held in state mental hospitals. If my story were to help free people, I'd say my life has been worth living. Oh, I value joyful moments in and of themselves, don't get me wrong. It's just that I feel as if I'm supposed to help others in some way.

"But Jane, you have."

119

Well, that young woman in the state hospital who stayed put because people out and about aren't nice...so what could I do to make life better for her? What does our society need to experience? How do we help society, including people with '"chemical imbalances",' feel safe? How can we help everyone feel safe? I don't know the answer to that. I try to let go of hurtful things people have said to me. Maybe some people are mean or stupid. It's not always about me. Bill Clinton said something once about how society should be ashamed, not the mentally ill.

It has taken me years to learn about myself, and it's still touch and go. I'm still learning. I'm always living with uncertainty, and maybe that's particularly why I believe in God.

The great thing about Branson, though, is that I worked so hard, and I mean hard, that it somewhat put my disorder in its place. I kept it under my thumb. I had one lengthy experience where my job "was the luxury of being more the focus", not my disorder. It was a great thing for a while. I even thought that maybe I had in some way leveled out and that my severe symptoms were gone for good.

Looking back, I think it might have been the 10-14 hour days that helped me sleep and, as I said, setting my own schedule. I mean, I struggled some, but I did very well. People thought I was brilliant, the best. From my end of it, that's hard for me to comprehend. I struggle in ways that I guess people don't see. Most people are aghast, amazed and appalled when they find out about my disorder. I'm not much of a stereotype. There's that word again.

Going back to spirituality, if I must, there were some things that really got my attention, things that helped me know there is some higher power, some greater order or sense that explained things. One day, I had a headache. I never had headaches. Carl and I didn't even have aspirin at home. So on my *way home from work, I stopped and bought aspirin and took two.*

When I got home, Carl hadn't gone to work. He said that he had a headache. I gave him two aspirin, and he went to bed. The next morning, he was performing in a theater. I had seen his show, and I hardly ever watched him perform by then. That morning, though, I felt concerned about how he was feeling, and so I went to the show. He was wrapping things up in his last couple of songs, and he was missing words. I had never seen him do that. Then it occurred to me, just a thought: he's had a stroke.

I ran and got my truck and drove to the back of the theater and went straight to triage with Carl. He seemed numb. He had had a stroke, and two main things were damaged: his short-term memory and his peripheral vision. The aspirin had stopped any further damage from occurring. It touched us deeply, Carl and me.

We did another album together after that. It was part of his rehab, so to speak, because I was determined that Carl would get back what he lost. I told him that making that album was better than sex. He told me he was glad he didn't have to choose. This was a gospel album, and he knew I was very serious about recording it. It meant everything to me that we did that one, much more important to me than all of the others.

Carl and I did nothing in the right order. We lived together before we knew each other. We were together six years before we got married. And sadly, we got divorced when we still loved each other. I'll always love him; he'll always have a place in my heart. I'm getting ahead of myself, though. Have I confused you, Carolyn?

"No, not really."

Not really? Okay.

Jane grows quiet.

I'm old. I'm old enough to see that I have never had what I wanted for myself. My life has never gone as planned, as wished. My life has been wrapped around my disorder. It's been that way since I was 16 or 17 years old. I rock-climbed in high school. One of my coaches was a climbing guide. Whenever we made it to the top, it was an amazing feeling. I wish I could feel that with my disorder. You know, Carolyn, I think I can, and I don't think I'm that far off.

When I ran in the Boston Marathon at age 16, I hopped a plane to Boston, ran it, and took a bus back to school. I got suspended for missing school, but back then, I really was on top of the world, so in control of myself. I used to think, okay, my life is a marathon, keep going, keep trying unless you need to quit. Quitting life is really scarey. I've been that way only a couple of times.

"Suicide?"

Yes, Carolyn, suicide. And I'd say that the worst was just a few years or so ago. It seemed that my pain would never end, but mainly that I could barely take care of myself. I saw no light at the end of that tunnel. No light at all, and I considered saying good-bye to this world. I mean, I was immobilized.

"What helped?"

Getting a part-time job as a tech and telling my parents how I felt.

Maybe my life is what Dr. Jobson said it is. Dragging an anchor, being a heroine. Will I ever reach the other shore? Carolyn, there are moments when I tell myself to hang on, that time helps. Like that TIME magazine while I waited to be admitted to a hospital, right out of jail. Jail can help. There are times when I wish I were in jail, because it narrows my world and contains me. Sadly, it had become a comfort zone, as have psych units and driving around at night.

And as I've said, Dr. Jobson told me to find the islands:

122

good people, good moments. For me, that would be moments in
time when I feel minimal symptoms. Even if things are awry all
around me, I live for those moments when I feel at peace. So I tell
myself to try to get through any given moment. You never know
when a good moment is on the rise. It's worth waiting for and
trying to make it happen.

And you know, I'm better at pain than triumph. I'm
comfortable on the bottom rung, major number one
underachiever, used to tough stuff, not ease and praise. How
many people worry that the stress of planning a wedding might
make them psychotic? How many people sleep in the closet just
from being so overwhelmed in any number of ways? Well, that's
what I've needed to do at times, times when I was sick. But if
God, by some miracle, wanted me recognized, I'd have no choice.
Have you ever tried to run and hide from God? He has an
advantage, I think. When it comes down to the bottom line, what
He says goes. Maybe He just thinks He knows what's best. I sure
would like to talk with Him about that.

I don't know what to say; a sadness comes over me.
Jane and I sit in silence. I still don't know everything that
has happened to her these past few years. It must have been
awful. She starts to cry quietly. We sit for many minutes.

"So what happens if you're ever recognized for a job
well done? I mean, you've done well at many things."

I'll deal with it, but doing mental illness well is not
valued in our society. It's that simple. Joy and freedom are plenty.
And it's been a long time since I've had someone say 'really nice
job'. Can you imagine someone saying that to a mentally ill
person who is doing well? Now that, I'd like to see.

Jane looks at me and laughs. She never holds a gaze
with me, never looks into *my* eyes.

"Jane, is it hard to look at me? It seems that way..."

Carolyn, connections are tough. It's hard to talk about this stuff. Imagine this, Carolyn. Imagine being in a hospital for life, looking out a window smudged with grime. Just rocking in a chair...and thinking underneath somehow that I would miss you.

I'm starting to understand this difficulty that unfolds. When can she say it's all okay, stand tall and be understood? Jane needs to see the light that she shines on others. She needs to step outside of herself and see how great she is. And maybe if she has to change meds again, it won't be such a nightmare. She's getting better and better at making good transitions happen, better at putting her foot down with doctors. Maybe the world will understand that, if she's out of pocket for a brief time, she's simply taking care of herself.

And yet what if she runs into medication trouble again and she's unable to get back to 'herself'? What would Jane say about someone in that predicament?

You've just got to keep trying, looking for a window.

"You need to know that you matter. No matter what." Jane smiles, but her eyes look to the floor.

Thank you.

Helplessness for a professional should never come easy.

CHAPTER THIRTEEN NO CONTROL

How do I tell people what I'm going through?

September 4, 2009

I'm feeling sad for Jane. It seems she'll never have that peace of mind she might feel without her disorder. Who knows, maybe she will, someday. She told me how she feels some sense of peace when she's got her sleeves rolled up and sweat on her brow. Why does that not surprise me?

Her next contact:

I think I wanted Carl to get better more than he wanted it. He seemed discouraged. We read, did word games, went grocery shopping, anything to challenge his mind. We played catch and tennis and basketball. He improved considerably in spite of a bleak prognosis.

However, something in him changed. He wanted to move back home. I didn't. I told him that I couldn't just up and leave, what about our bills. I said I'd need to get my counseling license changed over to Tennessee and line up a job. But he wouldn't stay. I really don't know what happened. I was numb. It was all just a blur. He told me that he couldn't stay a day longer in Branson. I was hurt, afraid, and angry, not to mention alone. I was at a loss as to how he was feeling, lonely, I would think, with me at work all day. I encouraged him to start playing again, but he just seemed really down. He left.

Once Carl was gone, guys who lived in the RV park knocked on my door incessantly, all for the wrong reasons. It was distracting and downright scarey. A center counselor named Karen, whom I greatly admired, knew what was going on, and she told me I could move the RV onto her land. I drove the RV out into the boondocks where she lived, and we became good friends.

Carl and I visited some over the next year. I guess we both felt that we'd let each other down. I thought about the hours we worked so we could have a roof over our heads, and the love we shared. But something had changed. I wanted to go to a marriage counselor, and he didn't. That hurt. I knew that I would always love him. I cried throughout our divorce process.

If everything really does happen for a reason, like our divorce, it spared him the agony of going through these past several years with me. Maybe he has a better life with a new wife. Several months after things settled, I called his aunt and said, "I just have one question, just one. Is Carl happy? I mean, is he?" She said yes, he is. "Thanks, I just needed to know." I got off the phone, and finding myself crying, I knew they were tears of both gratitude and relief.

***

September 10, 2009

I'm getting over the shock of Carl's departure and where it's left me. At least I'm busy. I'm not capable, some people say, of understanding what good things I've done for others – alcoholics, addicts, poor people, families, any clients, staff. I guess I don't comprehend the influence I can have, the power of helping people to the next level. The staff and I carry the actual services at the center to a level that I'm proud of, and what a staff! However, the work is just something in front of me to do, something good, something thoughtful. And once again, the staff are amazing, so trusting. They do everything I ask and make great suggestions. We are quite the team.

My parents come to visit, and they sing out gratitude that I'm divorced from Carl. They're angry with him. They worry that I'm left in Branson with no family there. I tell them it's okay. I tell them I have a job to do and that I have several friends. Then the bomb drops.

My parents and I are sitting in their motel room, and my dad asks me why my jaw is moving uncontrollably. One of my relatives had that problem when she was alive. My heart sinks, as I know what's going on. I cannot ignore it. I admit that I've developed tardive dyskinesia. I am so angry. Have I not gone through enough?

I tell my parents that I'll go to my doctor. I worry that it's permanent or will get worse, no matter what. I'm already thinking that I'll have to change medications, and there's no telling what that holds in store. I say goodbye to my parents and tell them that I'll call them every day and check in.

I'm sitting in the waiting room. I see an internist many miles outside of Branson who has prescribed the meds I've been on for a long time. He observes the twitching and jaw moving. He switches me to a newly-released antipsychotic.

The switch is clearly abrupt, and he has no idea how sick I can get. I, myself, have partly forgotten how bad things have been for me when it comes to psychosis. However, I do ask him if I can go in the hospital, and he says I'll be fine. How often I hate that word.

I'm sitting in a local pharmacy, waiting to get the script filled and in serious denial, all while being nervous, of what this might mean. I grieve the loss of my old antipsychotic. It has kept me out and about instead of in a state hospital. It's my comfort zone. I'm scared.

I sit down with Karen and explain the problem. She knows, like most people, that I've been on call 24/7 for close to ten years, and that I often go to work at 5:00 a.m. (I always went to bed very early.) I don't want to freak her out with the schizophrenia end of things, so I tell her that I have a bipolar disorder. I tell her that I'm switching meds and am not going to work so much. She's really cool about it all and asks if I want to move into her house, which I do.

I start on this new neuroleptic. It knocks me out like a light. And it feels as though my IQ has shot to the moon. Some of those people in psych units told me my IQ couldn't get any higher. Well, it has. When I look at myself in the bathroom mirror, I am hugging the sink for dear life. This isn't mania. This is a glimpse of who I might have been. It's so powerful that I almost can't stand it. I had no idea how far below my potential I'd been, not to mention set-backs and restarts.

I get the flu and lie in bed for a week. What is the flu, and what are my symptoms? I've always thought that depression and the flu were one and the same. My days and nights flip flop. I want my old medication back, but I can't do that.

A couple of weeks go by, and I see that I can't do my job as well as I had been doing it. I tell my boss that I am going to resign. I tell him that I want to go into private practice, that it's beyond time for me to leave, that I've done what I can do. He doesn't want me to quit. How do I tell people I'm ready to go, regardless of my health problem? I feel exhausted, although I'm sleeping better than I ever have. I can't seem to adhere to any kind of schedule, whatever that would be. I'm suddenly flying a jet while I've been accustomed to a small prop plane.

Christmas is approaching. I string Christmas lights in my room and keep my door closed. Karen doesn't say anything yet. I notice that my meds are running out, both the lithium and the new drug. I call my doctor, and it's an answering machine. He's on vacation for two weeks, something he didn't even tell me. What now? His answering machine says to go to an ER or call 911 in an emergency, but I'm not admission material, says the local hospital. Why must people like me wait until our lives are ruined? Did he not leave anyone on call? Nope. Whose door do I *knock on?*

Nonetheless, I'm still the associate director, still able to focus, still wanting to resign. I'm walking down the hall, when a tech in front of me trips and falls to the floor. I help her up and ask what's going on. She tells me she needs to see a doctor but has no health insurance. She said she falls a lot, her feet just going out from under her.

I have the authority to hire and fire, and so I ask if she'd like to work full time and thus have health insurance. She sighs with relief. I tell her to go on vacation, and that I'll get her the insurance and that she must see her doctor asap. She says she's supposed to see a neurologist. I say to her, go.

I drive over eighty miles to set her insurance in place at our main office. Meanwhile, the tech calls me and says that she has to have an MRI. She calls after the test and says she has a tumor on her spine.

A couple of days later, she calls again and tells me she's going in for surgery. I go to the hospital where she's prepped for the surgery. However, they won't do her surgery, because she lives in Arkansas and not Missouri. I drive back to our main office and get that worked out.

I'm waiting with her, and she says, "Jane, if two more weeks had gone by, I would have been paralyzed from my waist down." I tell her I'll be waiting for her when she gets out of surgery.

I go to the rest room and lock myself in a stall and bawl my eyes out. What if I had done nothing when she tripped? I pull myself together and meet her parents. I talk some with them while flipping through a magazine.

The surgery is a success. I try not to cry. But I do cry, out of relief, and out of anger over how our country has so many people who are without insurance and who cannot get the medical help they need.

***

I'm angry, so angry, and I beg for relief but am so tired. Just plain tired, and tired of being me. I'm ready to die. I put my resignation letter in my boss's box and leave. I pack up all of my things and put my stuff in Karen's storage shed. Then everyone realizes that I'm gone. Karen has never seen me like this; she's trying to do her job; she doesn't know what to do. She watches me leave the center. She sees how upset I am. She gapes at the way I run my mouth. She doesn't see that my disorder is keeping me from being a bit more professional, a bit less agitated. I'm not myself, she sees that.

I make a lot of noise as I'm rearranging my room. Karen keeps going to work, and she becomes beside herself. She leaves me a note on the kitchen counter. It says my resignation has been accepted and for me to please tell her what on earth is going on. I feel like a real burden and leave. I sold the RV, so where do I go? I find a motel and settle in. I want nothing to do with anyone. I've resigned and am not responsible for any clients or supervisees. So I sit, alone in a motel.

There's a knock at the door. I've only ordered pizza once, so who could this be? Who is it? I ask through the door. Police, open up, a deep voice barrels back. My heart jumps to my throat. Not jail again, I think. I open the door. There stand a man and a woman, dressed in blue, their gold badges shining.

I stand there numb and speechless, helpless and exhausted. They ask to come in, and they check my motel room for weapons and/or drugs, I guess. There are none, of course. I finally say, look, I just want to be left alone. I'm trying not to cause any trouble, and I love the center. I'm waiting for my doctor, I say. They give me a business card and ask me who I might talk with. I tell them the supervisor who helped me get my counseling license.

130

I promise them that I'll go see her, which I do. I load all of my stuff in my truck and drive 30 miles to my supervisor's office.

She doesn't know what to say or do. I say thanks and leave.

I call my dad who says he wants to come to Branson and bring me home. I recollect our trip back home from college, and I tell him, no thanks. He seems angry over the phone, although he's probably really just scared. I can't deal with him. Strangers don't seem so emotional. I tell him I'll call him every few hours.

I sit in the motel room several more days. I haven't slept for almost two weeks. I lose touch with when to call the right people and what to say. I leave that motel and check in and out of others, thinking people are after me, thinking people are trying to kill me. I get countless key cards to motel doors, as it takes me too many tries to enter my rooms. I run out of credit on my credit cards and don't know what to do.

I drive toward Karen's, and my truck starts to rattle, then steam spewing from under the hood. I can't believe this. I pull over, get out and walk several miles to a gas station where I buy a lot of bottled water with cash. I walk back to my truck, pop open the hood, twist off a cap and pour. I'm hoping that works.

I make it to Karen's, but she's not home. Still tired, I'm bored and revved and decide to run a marathon. I run for hours in the woods, although it's been months since I've exercised. I'm running as fast and light as I did when I was 16 years old. My body is what it should be, seems like no lactic acid, but my mind is orbiting aimlessly somewhere out in the universe. I'm never correlated.

I go inside and hide in my closet. Then I weigh myself and see that I'm ten pounds lighter than one week ago. I venture out of my room and go to the refrigerator. The dishes are piled up in the sink. This is ridiculous, I think. I stack the pots and pans up on the counter and scoop them up in my arms.

I take them to the back door but see that I can't get it open with all the pots and pans. I set them down and open the door. Then I can't get them all back in my arms. I take one pot, walk onto the porch, and end up heaving every single one of them into the air. They each go sailing over the back fence and into the woods.

I turn on my Christmas lights and cry, thinking that Karen is going to kill me. Yep, she's going to kill me. I'm eating all the peanut butter. Please, no one knock on the door. It's right around Christmas, and I'm actually wishing Jesus or even just Santa would show up.

I camouflage my truck with tree limbs and shrubbery, thinking Karen won't notice I'm home. We'll see. The front door opens. Jane, she yells. Oops, guess not such a great job. I hold my breath. She comes in my room and sees me holed up in the closet. I've been worried sick, she says. Let me help you, Jane.

I can't believe this. She says, "I didn't know at first. I'm sorry. Let me help you." Well, it's a bit late for that, I say. Can you please leave me alone? I ask, Pleeease? She walks out of my room, and I prop my feet up against a wall in the closet, still able to look at my Christmas lights. They look like stars in some vast unknown.

Karen comes back. Where's a skillet? she asks. Oh-oh. Does it really matter? I say. Well, where are they? she asks again. I'll go find you one, I say. I march my butt out the back door, down the patio stairs and make a running start trying to clear the fence. I get my shoelaces caught in the weeds I should have mowed, plow into the fence and bounce backward. What the heck are you doing? Karen asks. I'm trying to get you a freaking skillet! I yell.

Come back in, she says. Come in the house. Come in the

damn house. Come in the bleeping house. Have you talked with my parents recently? I ask, because you sound just like them. No, I haven't, and where's my toaster, did you throw that out, too? Now that would just be plain stupid, I say, throwing away a brand new toaster. It's out in the shed. Why? she asks. Oh, I don't know, I say, I don't know. Karen looks tired and, for once, uncertain as to what to say or do. Let me take you to the hospital, she says. I say, forget it. I already tried that, anyway. They said I'm not admit material. Material!

Karen goes to her room. I tiptoe toward her door and hear faint crying blending in with the TV. Is Karen on TV, I wonder? I remember me being on TV last year, in a spot about our center, when I was doing better than ever. I go back to my room. All night, I am still. Then it's early morning.

Karen leaves for work in the dark. I hear her pull out of the driveway. I stand up, and I think there are people in the house. I hear them whispering. I see their shadows move. I spend at least an hour as a detective, making my way to the other end of the house with great precision in my stance and movement. The people are gone, all except my partner who covers for me until I say "clear."

Once daylight arrives, I retreat to my closet and cry. I have a lot of cash on me but have no reason to buy anything. To me, it feels like 'game over.' The phone doesn't ring. No one comes to the door. I'm afraid to get the mail. I sit tighter than anything possible and wonder if maybe I should call 911. I wonder all day where I'm going to end up. Karen comes home and goes straight to her room.

With my sense unraveled, I can't wait any longer. It feels like suicide, but it's the right thing to do. I pick up my phone, and, as if pulling the trigger, I dial that short and sweet number: 911. Then I change my mind, but it's too late. The woman says she's sending someone out to check on me. I guess she meant it.

Soon, there are all kinds of lights flashing through the curtains. There's a knock at the door – the cops. I let them in just as Karen walks into the kitchen. What now? she asks. She writes something on a piece of paper and hands it to one of the officers. He sets the note down, and I grab it. I'm not on drugs! I holler. The note says: bipolar.

God help me, I guess I'm going to jail. That's usually part of the mix. I start to cry. One officer wants to see my meds. My room is a mess, I say. I trip over my Christmas lights and wish the officer a happy holiday. I've been making a career out of waiting for my doctor. The cop says he's going to find me a better one. Better career or better doctor? I think the latter. I ask him to please try the yellow pages and hurry.

CHAPTER FOURTEEN TRYING TO GET "HOME"

Oh man, can you believe this — walls as thin as rice paper.

The cop follows me into the bathroom, and I tell him I have no refills. I hand him the prescription bottles. Empty. He makes a call on his phone. Will you go with me to the hospital? he asks. I start to cry. Annoyed with me, Karen says, Jane, I've got to go to work tomorrow, you don't. I shoot her a look. Karen, how could you, how could you say that? I ask. She doesn't understand my life, what's this 'having to go to work' crap, and I cry alone, sobbing and shaking. She goes to get dressed.

An ambulance pulls into the gravel driveway. I usually go to jail first, I say. What's the problem, low on funds? I ask sincerely. Will you get in the ambulance? they ask. No, I say, still crying. Karen comes back in the living room. Get in the ambulance, Jane, just get in the ambulance.

Oh Karen, I see what's expected of me at this point, like I have a choice. You called 911, she says. Well, I didn't know it was going to be a production, you aren't helping. Just go back to bed, I tell Karen.

She tells the cop she'll follow them to the hospital. A parade? I ask. Great, I knew it. Thank God, the guy in the ambulance is nice and calm. Sorry for the trouble, I say. We pull into a hospital. I'm escorted to triage. I know the nurse. Everyone knows me from work — some legend, I think. You do a good job, Mark, I say to him who I know well over the phone. Bet you never thought you'd meet me like this. I feel so embarrassed, if I feel anything. He smiles as he takes my blood pressure.

It's all very confusing. I think that Karen is going to be my roommate in the hospital, and I pitch a fit, saying she's abusive. Then I realize that I think anyone who cares is abusive. Most people who care about me tend to yell, cuss and then get me very worked up.

Another nurse takes me around the corner. She ushers me into a room where the light is dim and the walls are gray. The colors I see aren't there, but they move about like molecules. Karen follows us in, as I hop up on the table. I hop way higher than needed, and I land with a thud on my elbow. Ouch. We're alone.

What year is it, Karen? I ask. No, what month is it? It's December, she says. Are my parents still alive? I ask her. Yes, they are, she says softly. I didn't even use your toaster, and I'll buy you a new bunch of skillets, I say. Man, you need a bunch of stuff, Karen. I'm going to make a lot of money someday, and I'll buy you a bunch of stuff. You watch me, I'm going to make a lot of millions of dollars and retire you out with a monster of a bank account. You deserve it. Shh, she says. Karen's seventeen years older than me but looks one hundred. It's all my fault, all my damn, bleeping...

Sorry about the commotion, I say. We're good, Karen says. You can go, I say. I'll be okay, you've got to go to work tomorrow, I say, tears running down my cheeks, and I don't. I wipe my nose on my arm, snot everywhere.

Karen says she does need to go, it's 3:00 a.m. by then. I whisper thanks, but she's already gone. The door closes heavily. I hop down and peep out the door. I see an orderly and hop back up too high again on the table, lie back and hit my head with a thud. For the first time in weeks, I feel safe enough to doze.

***

It's morning, although I don't know how many days have passed. I'm in a bed in a room with a window. My feet touch the cold linoleum floor. I peer out the door. There's a guy with a name

136

badge on his shirt. Hey, can you tell me where I am? I ask. I get oriented as best I can, realizing I'm in a psych unit in a town several hundred miles away. Is this lock down? I ask. Yes, he says. Good, no one can get to me, I say. He sort of chuckles. It doesn't bother me; I just want to feel assured about my safety. There are some lunatics out there, I say. You're fine, he says. How do people who say that know that?

Later that day, I see a psychiatrist. She's kind and tells me what meds she is going to try. Can you put me on what I was on before I ran out? I ask. She agrees to do so. I try so hard to come in for a landing. I do all the groups and activities and eat like no tomorrow. I sleep as if I were normal, but I'm still revved and thought-disordered. I want to stay on that unit forever. People are nice to me. However, I know I'm going to have to go back into the world where my well-being is touch and go. I bet I don't collect $200 this time around. Have I ever?

After two weeks, time's up. I have to present a plan to the staff, a plan concerning my departure and future. I tell my dad not to come get me. I'm going to do this Jane's way, and if you can't handle that, then don't be calling me, I tell him. I ask about taking a bus home. The bus leaves at 8:00 p.m., and it goes within 15 miles of Karen's home. Home, what's that? I figure I'll take the bus and then walk the rest of the way. How did my plan get approved? I might have told them I have a ride.

I put clothes on over my scrubs, another souvenir to go with my million dollar orange jumpsuit and PASS plaque. I'm going to frame these clothes some day. Maybe I'll iron them first. I have a plastic bag for my belongings. The director gives me a backpack at the last minute, along with some reading glasses. Over this past year, my vision has become compromised. So, I'm ready to go. I say goodbye to everyone, including a client I had who was in Drug Court.

137

He asks me if I came in to detox. I say, No, meds. He says good luck and gives me a hug. Look, I still have the wrist band you gave me, he says. He holds his arm up and reads the imprint on the rubber: Courage. We always had contests at the center where the clients could win wrist bands. I smile, walk to the door and take a deep breath. This isn't going to be easy, I tell myself. There's a little sane person in me trying to get out, and she's praying like hell. I'm nowhere near ready to go. Surely, everyone knows that.

An older gentleman gives me a ride to the hospital front door. We're on the elevator, and I wonder why the psych unit always seems to be on the top floor. If we jump out a window, we won't be coming back. Too late to jump, although my aftercare plan seems suicidal enough.

In the elevator, the man says something really interesting to me. He says, it's an honor to know you. I say to him, same back to you. Then we're quiet. I ask, do you know me or something? He says, everyone knows you, Jane, everyone. You've done so much good for people. Well, that's good, I say, I'm glad to hear that. Still, I'm a bit confused, because I never did get out much when I was working at the center. Oh well, I say, it's not like people send me flowers. Maybe that's best, I say, you know, just kind of quietly slipping out the back and leaving things as they are. The elevator door opens. A grand ceremony, and all taking place in an elevator. Thank you, he says. No, thank you, I say.

Ready for the next leg of my journey (phew), I hop in a cab, and the lady driver tells me about her kids, how proud she is of them. That's so awesome, I think. I tip her a lot, and she first refuses it. Buy your kids something, I say. I get out at a convenience store and walk to the counter to buy a bus ticket.

There are no buses going there, a lady at the counter tells me. You need to catch a bus here, she points on a map, and then *get another bus, there. She points again. Her nails are long and painted. And the bus you want will be here at 12:40 a.m., if it's on schedule. Someone has made a mistake, and it's not me.*

I could take a cab back to the hospital and start over. No, too much paperwork and no more insurance coverage. I could get a motel room. Things are much more stressful out and about than they were on the unit. I realize that I should still be inpatient for another month. Again, what is with it with insurance? Things are jumpy in my vision, and it's not about wearing glasses. What am I going to do? I wonder if I look like a psychiatric patient. Are my scrubs showing through? Oh, I don't know. I look down my front. Shit, the tag goes in the back.

I walk outside and try to figure out what to do. There are two guys by the gas pumps, smoking. Now that's intelligent. One of them is buying pot, and they are laughing. At least it's not a school night. I go back inside. A cop walks in. Oh man, I hope he's not after me. I try not to feel startled, and that's not easy. It's a major effort. I go back to the counter and tell the lady I'll take that 12:40 a.m. bus to the closet stop to where'd you say, Joplin?

I'd just like to get home, I say, feeling like Dorothy and Kansas. Joplin, yeah, a ticket to Joplin, please, m'am? So far their maps seem updated every six hours, and it looks as if I won't be going straight to Springfield. Acceptance, I say 10 times under my breath.

I sit for hours. People come and go. People buy beer and coffee and donuts, yuk. I blow my nose on toilet paper from the bathroom, over and over. My parents don't know where I am. I'm thinking that, if they were to miraculously pull up about now, I'd break through a car window to get in. But missing my parents quickly becomes a non-issue. I know they won't be pulling up.

It's 1:00 a.m. I'm sweating, and I leap to my feet and run outside. Wrong bus, wrong damn bus. I sit down on the curb and somewhat wish I had jumped out that window on the unit. How am I going to get through the next couple of days? 'One minute at a time' tricks me into believing I can do it. Another bus shows up. Please, be for me. It is.

I get a seat in the front next to a large woman who has a cold. I try melting into the window as she falls all over me. Hi, I say. The bus pulls out, and a couple of hours go by. I am suspended in sheer prayer. It was simple: God help me. I get off the bus and wonder if I'm even going to make it back to life at least close to how I once knew it. I have my doubts.

I see my next bus isn't leaving until mid-morning of the following day. I realize I can't sit up that long. I hail a cab in my semi-reality. I ask to go to a motel in a nice area of town. Why he's passive-aggressive, I don't know, as he drops me off in front of a strip club. There's a motel right behind it. I just want to hug a mattress. I walk in and ring the bell. A guy finally approaches the front desk, wearing a t-shirt and boxer shorts. I get a room key. It takes me, honestly, twenty minutes to find the number on the door that matches the room key.

Success! I walk in. It smells like smoke. I flop on the mattress as I've done so many times in my life, in so many different situations. I take my meds and lie there in the dark. It's rather quiet, and I try not to cry. My bed starts to vibrate. What's going on? I look to see if it's one of those massage beds, but I didn't put any quarters in a slot. I roll over. My teeth are humming. I hear noises. I lie ever so still. I hear moaning and...groaning. Oh man, can you believe this – walls as thin as rice paper.

I feel so defeated and out of pocket that I try calling numbers scribbled on the wall. One phone number is a freebie, phone sex...call Zelda? Hmm. I'm curious, so I call and ask her why this job? She starts right in, Baby, I've got you in my

140

arms...You do not, I say, and I'm thinking, she's as crazy as I am. Do you need help? I ask her. I'm thinking more along the lines of phone counseling. She thinks I'm a turn on. Who knows what she means! I hang up, somehow recognizing that I'm getting distracted and am probably not going to get many good suggestions from her or my neighbors. How can anyone sleep? Oh, Jane, I tell myself, for once, stop being so naïve.

I get up and march back to the front desk, my adrenalin overriding the sedation of my meds. I get my money back and call for another cab. I get in and tell the guy, look, damn it, a nice part of town. He drops me off in front of a hospital next to a motel. Close enough. This time, I walk in a room, lock the door and head to use the phone. No, it's the middle of the night. Leave the phone alone. I lie on the bed and either pretend or really think I'm on a raft in the middle of an ocean. I think it's the latter, oh well, nothing much new about that these days. Daylight approaches, taking forever but never long enough.

I'm reluctant to return to the bus station. It's all such an ordeal. I call Karen. She says to let her come pick me up. I fold. It's time to appreciate all she's done for me. We drive home in silence. We get part of the way home, and I tell her I'll be gone as soon as I find a place to stay. She quietly tells me fine, if that's what I need to do. If I have ever fished for answers, it'd be then. Fine is not the answer I was looking for. Have I told you how I hate that word?

I light up a cigar that I bought at the convenience store and puff and puff but don't inhale. Wanna' try, I ask Karen. What I want is for you to put that out, she answers. Well, one of the social workers said a big fat cigar is good for the soul now and then. Just let me finish it, on account of my poor soul really needing help these days, I say.

Do I need to take you back to lock down? she asks. I shoot

her a look. Well, I'm just asking, she says. Nope, that clear as day is a threat, and I toss the cigar out the window. What a waste, I tell her. Silence the rest of the way to her home.

***

I call a county clerk because I missed my court date for rear-ending a lady's car two months earlier. They have a warrant out. I go immediately to court and pay my fine. They promise they'll pull the warrant. I go see my doctor only for scripts. How was your vacation? I ask. Oh, we had a wonderful time skiing, he says.

Yeah, me, too, I say. Our conversation is pressured. I am so angry that I just decide to keep my mouth shut and not get wound up.

I drive home and go to my room. I trip over clothes and Christmas lights, and I weigh myself: 104 pounds. My ribs stick out. I try to eat. I force myself to eat. My sleep is fitful. I have a long way to go. I work on getting money for short-term disability. Karen tells me that some people think I'm crazy and never want to see me again. Great.

I drive to Wal-Mart. It's brand new. I leave the parking lot and am pulled over by a cop. Damn those flashing lights forever. He tells me I used the wrong exit. I was going the right way, though, wasn't I? I ask. He takes my license and comes back, asks me to step out of my truck and says there's a warrant out for my arrest. He cuffs me, and I ask, what now?

He tells me that he'll take me in to one county, and the next day, they'll move me to another county, then it's the weekend, and then I'll see the judge some time next week. I get the idea that it's over that warrant they said they "pulled". I beg him to call someone. I tell him I can't go that long without my medication, that I just got out of the hospital. He drives toward the justice center. It's quiet except for the terror ringing through *my mind.*

I sit in the back seat with my hands behind my back, thinking my relationship with cops is too much at times. He says to me, who can I call? I say, the county clerk. He says, tell me the number. I close my eyes and see the Rolodex card and tell him the number. He calls. He turns the car around right as we enter the parking lot. Sorry, ma'am, it's their mistake. I'm used to working with liars, he says. I don't lie, I say. I may be crazy, but I don't lie.

He takes me back to my truck where a tow truck has arrived, and he pops off the cuffs. The cop tells me I'll have to pay for the tow truck, but I'm free to go. He says forget the ticket and go out the other exit from now on. I go to pay the tow truck guy and see it's a client who went through the center. He's sober and happy. He gives me a hug. Everywhere I go, that happens to me. He doesn't make me pay him.

I'm determined not to relocate, something seemingly inevitable that I did in my past. I'm going to stand my ground. I discover that I can go on short-term disability for three months, but what a headache to get a check. I'm still slipping in and out of a few mild symptoms but am released back to work after three months, part-time. I'm also facing many distractions from knowing that a lot of people think very poorly of me. However, I stay focused in my work, which has much less emotion than sitting around does. After three months, I set up an office for a part-time private practice.

A lot of people call, and I'm in business. I work four hours per day and rest in my free time. I have a contract with one of the courts, and they like what I'm doing. Dealing with clients is easy. It's everyone else I have trouble with.

I write apology notes to people I called in the middle of the night and people I spouted off to. People start hearing how what

143

happened to me involved medication changes, and most of them ease into that reality. It gives them some sense of control over the vast and frightening unknown. Explanations sometimes go a long way. It's nice to see that a lot of people meet up with some understanding and a hands-on gain of knowledge, even if it's at my expense.

A lot of clients from the center either ask if I'll be their therapist, or they want to ask me what happened. Everyone in the area knows, and some people are kind. A few are cruel. Some people want to learn, and others choose to be ignorant. Some people are hateful, and others are loving. It's sometimes hard to know just what kind of day or week or month or year or decade any given person might be having. So in my book, it pays to show kindness, a simple (but why so difficult?) way of being in this world.

CHAPTER FIFTEEN TRYING AGAIN

Get back on that bronco, and ride it 'til it throws you.

September 24, 2009

"Come on in, Jane."

How's it going?

"Good."

Am I writing too much?

"Not at all."

Carolyn, what do you think? I mean, what do you think about me?

"You have a lot of tenacity. You do damage to your illness. I'd like to see you get even smarter, even tougher. I say that, because I think you can. And I'd like to see you put what you do into words for others to use. Get things down to a fine art."

Fine? Ha, ha, ha, Carolyn, but there's nothing all that funny. I've got this thing for life! But you know, I'm gaining on it. I'm learning. I'll start thinking about some kind of a workbook or something.

I used to go outside with shorts and a T-shirt on and sit in the snow for hours. I used to go in my parents' garage and sit on the concrete and stare at my feet for hours. Someday I'm going to paint my toe nails. I think that'd be fun. You know, Carolyn, I've given it all I've got.

"And then some. Jane, I think you have something major to offer, really.

And tell me now, what exactly would that be?

"The way you teach yourself. The way you do things...the way you decide...the way you think. Hmm, it's your hope for change. People have hurt you, and you hope

145

they change. I know it's hard."

Isn't that self-serving? For me to want people to change? I mean, come on, Carolyn. Think about it.

"No, it's not, not completely. You hope they learn. You have hope for other people's sake. Forgiveness. Acceptance. You have hope that people become more at one, you know, helping one another. Showing some understanding, or at least trying to."

Well, there are a lot of mentally ill people whom I know that have died in the throes of close-mindedness. I know because I have brushed up against it.

It isn't easy out and about. We have to hang in there and focus on staying centered, take the bull by the horns as if it's our last breath...and realize that a lot of people don't get it. There are people who wish we were dead, that we didn't exist. There was a time when the answer was hysterectomy. There was a time when I was angry my parents had me. You've got to be really tough. It's our world, too. We belong here.

The stigma is worse than the illness. I am guessing that my toughest battle has yet to be fought. It's going to be very hard having a lot of people know, if things go that way. It's human nature for people to see only 'mental illness' in a person when you tell someone you have one. And the fear from not understanding makes us all crazy. That's why we need to unite.

"I guess this is just a wish, Jane, but I wish people could see your life's truth."

My wish is that a lot of wrongs be righted in one fell swoop. I don't bank on that, though. Things take time. However, if a lot of people do read my story, then so be it. I don't want it all to be about me. It's not about me. And it's not even all about mental illness. It's about people. If I have to, though, I'll learn how to respond to everyone knowing. Maybe I'll wear a T-shirt that says 'I'm on the right meds'. And if not, my T-shirt will be turned inside out, and I'll put the tag in the front.

Jane smiles. I smile. She tells me all about her ride back from the hospital. I lose all control and laugh until it hurts.

Yeah, hilarious, thanks a lot. Can we get back to reality here?

"Sorry, Jane, but it's the way you explain things." Jane plows ahead.

I think I need to wipe away the shame that society has smeared all over me. I need to be above that. If I carry shame about myself, I carry it about others, too. I know there are so many great people who get tangled up when trying to step out or when their illness puts them front and center. Like me! It's about more than me being a person.

Carolyn, I'm a doctorate-level therapist, and I take that very seriously. It brings a host of potential, additional criticism – or higher praise. It's more complex, but you know, to my knowledge, I've never harmed a client. If so, no one ever told me. And we're talking 22 years of serving people in a variety of mental health services. Being ethical is of utmost importance.

When I'm sick, I do have to get out of the way. I refer my clients and leave or get things worked out and return. That's the ethical thing to do, even if it costs me. Clients have to be referred, and they don't like that. However, people get sick. It hasn't happened all that often, three times in 22 years, and it's been costly to me when I leave a job. It means, at some point, I usually start back on the bottom, so to speak. And it usually takes a while to get completely well. What angers me most is that, when my doctors are negligent, it affects not just me but my clients and co-workers.

What's helped me is that I've told my professors; I've

147

called licensing boards for advice; I've asked Dr Jobson to call whomever I need him to call; I've been a really good consumer with doctors and therapists. I'm encouraging people to do just that. It makes a difference. For example, if I have a question on a licensing application, I make a phone call.

Nonetheless, I need to swap in my shame for a bouquet of flowers or something that represents an understanding of mental illness and the dignity that, believe it or not, I've created just in trying. I close my eyes and see something beautiful amidst the horrendous pain. That beauty has to do with the way I've triumphed, the way I've tried. Winning is trying. I still have trouble seeing that, but it's there for me. And it's an understanding there for people to see, if they would look for it. People who are mentally ill can do what I do to have better lives. Some people don't even know what meds they're on. Some people stay at home and won't go outside. It's fear. Empowerment is one of the keys.

Whenever symptoms creep up on me, I want to hide. However, I try to face my symptoms head on, or at other times, I rest. Whatever I'm doing, if I start having trouble, I change things up – you know, do something different than what I've been doing. And I call Dr. Jobson.

All the while practicing self-talk. I guess I know how to endure and face difficulty. Whatever it is about me, though, also involves being able to help others. I'm good at helping me, and I'm good at helping others. Probably contrary to the stereotype, I'm very strong and can withstand a lot of stress. Of course, it depends on the nature of the stress. I can work long, hard hours, but it's not easy being micromanaged.

Jane pauses. I wonder if she sees herself as a beautiful person, illness or not. What was it she said about the patients in state hospitals, that they have elegant

148

minds...

"So what happened to you in Branson?"

I went home to visit my parents, and I tried to reassure them that I was okay. I was doing well in Branson, but I couldn't sleep at all when I was in Knoxville. I was trying to balance myself every moment. I couldn't shut my thoughts off, which got in the way of my sleep. On my drive back to Branson, I'd had it with trying and was afraid of getting psychotic. I'll pick beer over psychosis just about any day. I drank two tall beers and was pulled over by a cop. He took me to jail. I spent two nights in jail, had nightmare symptoms while awake, and I was scattered, disoriented.

My parents were furious with me and scared of my being in the system. I was let go after two days, and I drove on to Branson. I told Karen that I got a DUI. I thought she'd throw my things out or something. She gave me a big hug. It opened up conversation between us. She, being a substance abuse counselor, could relate to my DUI, and her compassion was unreal. She and I were back on really good terms, and over a DUI!

"Maybe people just don't always know what to say. Maybe it's hard for the best of people to understand mental illness. How many people tour state hospitals, I mean, really, Jane."

Point taken. As we talked, Karen told me she had lost the best boss and friend she'd ever had when I changed meds. I was too preoccupied at the time to know that. She was hurt, angry and scared. And she felt she couldn't talk with me about it. She said I withdrew, like I had died, like something in me died. It took me a long time to catch up after three weeks of insomnia. What a true friend she has proven over and over. She is one of the most amazing persons I've ever known. She's strong; she cares; she is so close to God, closer than anyone I know, and I find that so incredible. She doesn't even swear anymore.

She has faced and triumphed over all kinds of difficulties, cancer twice, so many stressors, and she just keeps on going. She has been an amazing mentor to me. Actually, I'm in awe of her. When I moved in her home, I had a room on the far side of her house, and I never came out of my room, because I was in such awe. She told me I could come out, if I wanted. It took me a month to do so after she said that.

In any event, it was a long time before any doctor upped my medication. If I had had it in me to read, I would have discovered that the milligrams prescribed by the internist were way too low, that someone such as I needed much more.

Anyway, when I got back to Karen's, I was hanging on a shoestring. That whole trip to my parents and back was stressful. I closed up my practice, knowing I was going to move. I was having trouble finding someone who knew how to help me manage the medication. I stayed with it for a year. I'm glad I did.

I realized my dad wasn't going to live that much longer. It occurred to me that I should move near my parents.

The medication swap left me unable to recover fully. I could function, but I knew I could do much better. The lady I rear-ended was suing me. And with my DUI, there were the legal consequences. I knew I'd have to tell the counseling licensing board about that, and I would need to change my counseling license over to Tennessee. I also knew I needed to declare bankruptcy. All of this over a medication change!

I was overwhelmed. It isn't easy swimming against a current.

"I think it's amazing you stayed there a year."

I would have stayed longer, but seriously, I knew my meds were not being managed optimally, and there was just no help, it seemed. But you know, what's good is that a lot of people came around, and I did good work. But it was frightening for me. The psych unit where I stayed was great, but I didn't get what I needed as an outpatient with the exception of a really good therapist. The inpatient plan was to keep upping the antipsychotic medication.

I couldn't find any doctors who would do that. Maybe they were there, but I never found them. And I had stopped getting better. I saw some internists in the area who were no help, and I then started seeing a psychiatrist fifty miles away (the closest) and who, big surprise, wanted me off the new neuroleptic, when he should have simply upped the dosage. I'm so tired of doctors not seeing things the way they are.

No one seems to understand that I have a thought disorder. I have a disorder that is lodged seriously in the heart of schizophrenia. My thought disorder is chronic, daily. I have to take a very high dosage of an antipsychotic every day, for life. I've created a way of dealing with people in which I can ignore a lot of the symptoms, or they're treatable with meds. I'm way out there on the cutting edge in both psychiatry and psychology when it comes to functioning. And I understand the risks when it comes to tardive dyskinesia, but what life do I have when I'm forever psychotic without this medication? Fortunately, the new antipsychotic drugs have less chance of this side effect developing.

"The thing with you, Jane, is that...even when you're moderately disordered, Schizo-Affective Disorder does not come to mind. Not to me. Likely not to others. It doesn't fit you."

What, it doesn't fit me like a dress size?

"No." I laugh. "I just don't think people who have accomplished what you have would think you have such a severe and serious disorder. Do you think I understand how your upsets have occurred? Your doctors, three I think, and then the tardive dyskinesia. And when you're disordered a long time, it's hard getting well, and you've really had to face a limited career."

You do understand.

Jane pauses.

"I do know, and I'm sorry. You deserve so much more."

Sometimes I think that only my whole story allows people to see the full range of what a life can be. It's all true. There's this myth that I shouldn't be able to be exactly who I am – to have the illness I have, to be the person I am, to be the professional I am.

Surely this world should be ready for that. It saddens me to know that ignorance, close-mindedness, stupidity, arrogance and bias are killing a lot of people who could be happy and productive.

Here's one among many examples: I know clients who are petrified of psych units. I know therapists who seem to think we've killed someone by helping them be admitted. I'd be dead 10 times over without psych units. What are they there for? It's society that sends the horrible message about psych units. People get sick, they need a hospital, what's the problem? I know, because I really struggled with this issue.

"I hear you."

After resigning from my contracts and closing up my practice, I loaded up a U-haul and said goodbye to Karen. She didn't want me to leave at that point. I gave her a hug, and I was on my way. My dad wanted to fly to Branson and drive back with me. I threw a fit. I told him that we were going to be doing this my way.

Jane seems annoyed.

I made it to my parents' home, and I was very excited to see them. I called Dr. Jobson, and he got me right in. By then, I

152

was sleep-deprived and exhausted and feeling hopeless. I really missed Branson. My parents' reactions became a terrible burden. I heard my dad tell my mom that he didn't deserve having to put up with this, which devastated me, for countless reasons. I told him that he'd had the life he wanted, that I was the one who never had a break, he didn't live with what I have, he chose to have kids, and on and on. I saw so much stacked against me. So many things that I had to walk through to get a breath of air. I could maintain in Branson, but at my parents' new house, everything was unfamiliar. It stressed me in a way that actually even exacerbated my disorder.

Dr. Jobson upped my neuroleptic dosage. I told my parents I needed to get on long-term disability. At least I'd have some kind of income. I saw a lawyer who told me something astounding.

He said, "Jane, get back on that bronco, and ride it 'til it throws you." "Again?" I said, stupified. "How many times?" I stormed out.

I was sitting at a stop light, feeling like a mess, and then what the lawyer said made me laugh a little. And you know what? I took his advice. I forgave my dad but stayed stuck on 'how could you' for a good while. However, I think I actually passed Go this time and collected $200. Wow! My dad told me he was sorry for saying that, that it's rough for parents, he didn't mean what he said about me, he said it about my disorder.

I realized my dad's age had a lot to do with it. I will say this: when I came home, he sat down with me and said, "Jane, I'll hang in there with you as long as I can." That meant the world to me. He was saying, I think, that I was welcome in my parents' home.

He also told me something else. He said, "I know of no one who has accomplished as much as you. I see it, and I know it. And

I'm sorry that others don't see things the way they should."

It stunned me, because my dad has worked alongside the best physicians in the world. I said, "You mean, considering what I've been up against?" Because I think he's always been in denial. He said, "No, I'm talking about your education, the many hundreds of people who have really needed the help whom you've helped, and whatever it is you've done to help yourself. The way you, yourself, keep yourself afloat and keep trying even when you're medically mismanaged. I don't know how you do it." I said, "Wow, Dad, thanks." I think my parents know all kinds of things they don't tell me, as though they're afraid of saying something that'll get in my way.

"So, Jane, can you put that in the bank and make it count? What your dad said?"

Sometimes I can. I mean, he's not the only one who has said that. A lot of people in Branson said that when I went through the medication change problem. Anyway, things started ironing out. My insurance agent settled the wreck where I rear-ended that lady, meaning I didn't have to go to court.

I went through the consequences of my DUI. Then the executive director of the counseling license board called, of all things, and told me she appreciated my candor in the letter I sent in. I had written a letter saying I drank beer and shouldn't have and was addressing my issues surrounding the conviction. I found out that my license was never even suspended over anything and that no one had ever complained. I had handled things appropriately. She said that the board had voted for no consequences over my DUI, but don't let that happen again.

"Why didn't they let you off? Why couldn't they have taken the DUI off your record?"

A law prevents them from doing that. But for whatever reason, I was actually guilty for once. I did drink beer...Actually, *though, in jail, they did ask if I needed a hospital, and I said no. I did feel safe in their jail, comfort zone (a mattress, of course) and less complex than all that admit process, which is very stressful. Jail, they just take a photo and all, and that's it, then they leave you alone, pretty much.*

I'm trying so hard not to laugh. "So then..."

So then, as I was saying, I was soon free to transfer my counseling license over to Tennessee. I was still having trouble, although I could hold it together by trying too hard. My license has always been in good standing. Counseling boards are set up to protect people like me, who go through the right channels and do the responsible thing in times of stress or illness.

I first took two exams, which took a long time. There was a lot of waiting. The whole transfer took a year, and I have my counseling license to do clinical work here.

I had applied for a job as a tech at a treatment center and worked there for one and a half years, while I saved some money and waited to get my counseling license transferred. It gave me a chance to start sleeping and heal. I started out at the center working 20 hours per week; that was all that was available.

I must have done a good job at work, because once I had my license, I became the clinical director. I felt lucky just to wake up every morning and know who I was when I looked in the mirror. I worked very hard for the staff and those clients.

However, I wanted a job that was more like private practice, something outpatient. I wanted to work with clients with a wide range of issues. I still didn't have the money or clientele to set up a practice. I found an outpatient setting and worked there for almost one year. It was high-paced, but it helped me grow and even thrive.

Carolyn, it's worked out for me. Three years of a rough go to get where I am now.

"Three years?"

Three years here. And now I'm in a good group practice. I work with teens who are in foster care. And I have several clients who have major mental illnesses.

I sit in amazement and relief. So she's been busy establishing a job she loves, all while telling me her story. Jane has become stronger over time, while getting better sleep, while being herself. I start to cry, and I can't stop the tears. So I give in and let them roll and roll down my cheeks. Jane hands me a paper towel and points to my plant.

I was right about you, Carolyn. You're real. I love that about you. But what are you crying for? Tell me.

"I don't know. I've been sitting on the edge of my chair ever since I met you. It's been really hard hearing about what you've had to live with."

Carolyn, a lot of people live with what I've gone through. And a lot of people in this world have lived with much, much worse. Look at your history books. Look around you and stop sniffling.

"Yes, but I *know* you, and I've had a connection with you. You have wanted me here."

I know.

I've been *right here*. This has all been very real for me."

It's all been very real for the both of us. Carolyn, it's time for me to go.

"Wait a moment, Jane."

CHAPTER SIXTEEN GUNS AND THINGS

...it's too easy to pull the trigger.

Jane sits very still, and there's some kind of emotion between us that I cannot, for the life of me, explain. Maybe it's all in my mind. I feel a connection that I know will end, and it's making me a little crazy. Yet I've had questions in the back of my mind, as I've waited throughout her process, which I want answered.

I don't want to lose this moment because there has to be some spin-off of good that might guide her in the right direction and prevent her from mishaps. It might help her to talk with me just a bit more. Because even in her matter-of-factness, there's a world out there that she may not fully comprehend. I think she sees it, but it's as if it doesn't scare her. I don't want to see her hurt as she continues to improve. All I want is for her to be protected, prepared. And I want to know more about *her* plans for a book. Who's writing this so-called book?

"I want to know who you want to help. Who is your audience?"

Readers of my book? The project is yours. Anyone who can be helped by a book, great, but leave me out of it. Maybe teenagers, physicians, college students, parents, people with mental illness, family members, law enforcement, therapists, social workers, probation officers, addicts, women, men. Carolyn, it's fully up to you.

"So you still want me to make it public?

If you feel like it! Who else might I ask? No one else knows my story. Yeah, people know their end of it, they see glimpses. That's all it is, though. Yes, I want you to do whatever you think you should do with my writings and my chart and your perspective. I have no one else to ask, no one. And I guess you need to search in your heart and figure out if you're up for it.

"Which I am." I realize I'm grinding my back teeth when I say that. Only I'm not angry. I'm determined.

Carolyn, just follow your heart. I'm sure you'll do fine.

"Fine? Did you say fine?" Jane ignores me. We sit in silence for a minute or two. Maybe that's the best we each can do. I can't come up with any order in my questions.

I finally look at her and blurt, "Do you own a gun?" I take a quick breath, thinking it's the wrong way to ask how Jane protects herself.

What?

"How do you protect yourself? You know, mace, that kind of thing."

You said gun. So gun it is.

"I just worry about you. Some women carry protection..."

Well, this opens up a new line of questioning, doesn't it? No, I do not own a gun. I don't think I ever will. My, this does raise an issue, though. Obviously, you aren't mentally ill. Yeah, I'm a woman, and yeah, I'm alone a lot, but I'm also mentally ill.

"And?"

Well, should people like me be allowed to own a gun? I have thought about the guns and violence issue. I know what it's like to be me alone against a cruel world. I know the anger and hurt and fear I've felt. I've never been violent, though. I've never misused a gun.

When I was just turning 17 years old, I competed in cross-country skiing at a Junior National Competition. The Men's United States Biathlon Team was there. They were loaning all the juniors rifles, and it was a big recruiting-type operation.

158

*Biathlon for women was going to become an Olympic event, and
so one of the men loaned me his rifle and told me what to do. You
know, you ski five kilometers and stop and shoot and ski...and
shoot. It's hard, because you're breathing really hard when you
come in to shoot, not to mention you're carrying your rifle and
have to get all lined up and so on. Well, I had to hit ten targets,
and if you miss a target, you ski a penalty loop. Long story short,
I out-skied everyone – 15 kilometers, but the clincher was that I
hit all ten targets. Never fired a gun before in my life. So I was
very interested in this sport, and especially in pioneering an
endeavor to recruit women.*

*Then when I went out west for my junior year of college, I
trained with the Men's Team out there. They, too, loaned me a
gun. And when I became homeless and slept in my car, the gun
was actually in the back floorboard all during this time that I was
crazy and paranoid and spooked very easily. Yet I never thought
of using the rifle for anything except target practice at the range.*

"Gosh."

*Well, I returned the gun before I went to my sister's
graduation. Should I own a gun these days? I don't think I
would, even if I were perfectly normal. Where would I carry it –
my purse? It'd probably go off at the wrong moment. I'd probably
be looking for my car keys and blow a hole in my foot.*

"Well, you have to be careful."

She ignores me and keeps talking.

*I'd rather be shot than face having shot someone, hands
down. A gun would not be a good idea for* my *sake. The gun issue
is a non-issue for me. There are far more important things to
argue, like how words can kill. Every time someone shows
prejudice against the mentally ill with words, it's a step
backward. I believe, once again, love is the only way to fight fear.*

Maybe if I'd been a guy, it would be different. Maybe I'd

have shot someone. Maybe I'd have been shot. Maybe I'd have shot myself. I know two guys who have. So did my grandfather. Men have it rough. I think there's a double standard, men supposedly stronger than women. It's tougher on guys, mental illness, or so it seems to me.

Once again, Carolyn, I picked up a gun for the first time and nailed every target. And that gun was a real gun, but hurting someone or protecting myself never occurred to me. And I know I left it out of my story, but I have almost been killed – every page of my life, someone somehow, even unknowingly, has been working on the side of killing my spirit. It's what people carelessly say about the mentally ill. And ironically, there's more: People see my strength and sort of take things out on me, not knowing of my illness, thinking things don't bother me, that I'm very strong. I ignore a lot, but it's hard. Anyway, I have no plans to ever be in a situation of getting shot. But I've lived through far worse every day of my life. It feels that way.

Carolyn, when I was out west in college, I was smack in the middle of the schizophrenia part of my illness. It had really taken hold. But I was not suicidal. There have been two times when I have narrow-mindedly seen little point in a life like mine. It's too easy to pull the trigger. A gun is a serious issue for a lot of people.

"I understand. Sorry about how I asked about that."

No, it raised an important issue.

"Have you ever been suicidal when you've been seeing clients?"

No, but I know the feeling, and all I know to do that works is to see about hospitalization and say to clients, okay, see how you feel tomorrow, and keep saying that, all while trying to get to the bottom of it. As my dad said, there's no changing your mind if you kill yourself. And you know, I've made up my mind that,

160

in the worst situations, I don't want to miss anything. If there's a
miracle around the corner, I want to see it. I want to be there.
And you know, in our own ways, we are all miracles. All of us
are. We all need to believe that things can get better, because it's
true.

  And if someone needs a hospital, then so be it. I just hate it
for the many people who keep going round and round in psych
units or those who are in long term care who might experience
more freedom with the right kind of support. It's a tough pattern
to break, especially when the staff pass out so many perks, you
know, enable patients."

  Jane is dead serious in explaining that. I sit in
disbelief. I'm not sure what to do. "Do any of your
professional peers here know about you?"

  Not yet.

  "Any plans to tell someone?"

  Maybe. I mean, they'll know if this so-called book ever
gets off the ground.

  "What do you..." Jane interrupts.

  When it comes to all professionals, especially the ones who
know me, how would they respond to me, you know? I hope
they're supportive.

  Maybe you need some good friends.

  Yeah, maybe. I have a few.

  Jane smiles.

  My first time in one of the juvenile courts, some of the
lawyers who were involved sent me flowers (yep, it was a jolt),
and one of the attorneys thought I'd done a better job than any
mental health professional ever. Better at what, being nervous?

  When I was testifying, I told myself to be open with my
ideas and observations involving the family. I was on the stand

for what I think was over an hour, close to two. Question after question...but anything to help these kids.

In court, I try to help by answering questions so that the judge has enough information from me, hopefully objective, to then make the best decisions. I'm just a cog in the wheel, but I take it very seriously. I consider, in court, judges to be higher powers. I'm just there to try to help.

"That doesn't surprise me. But Jane, be good to yourself. Find people who can be good colleagues and friends to you."

There are many things I am never going to get. I guess I'm always going to have these awkward adolescent moments. I do, I feel like such a teenager. I often grow very, very fast, and it's really awkward for me.

If/when anyone I know reads my book or your book, how does one say hello? How does this all play out? I hope they talk with me again. I hope they know I'm just me, and I'm okay.

"Is that faith then?" I ask.

It's hope. I hope they understand and see the help I've provided and the ethics I've displayed. You know, not every job change has been over my illness. On many occasions, I simply saw jobs where I might be best equipped to do the most good I could do. With others, sometimes it's time to go.

Jane is quiet, as we sit in a new silence. I'm gripping the armrest of my chair. I glance at the clock. I know she's going to move on from me.

CHAPTER SEVENTEEN THIS LITTLE LIGHT OF MINE

Our lives always begin now.

October 8, 2009

I don't know when I will see Jane again. As for any book project, either hers or mine, she has no interest in recognition or money. She just asks that it's helpful and good, that it might help a few. I'll need to figure out how to get it published and how to contact her in the future – she told me to e-mail her the final draft. She said she fully trusts me and that she will not respond as to what she thinks of the final product. Jane told me that she doesn't want to get caught up in manuscripts, editors and publishers, but that she needs to stay on track with her health and job. I respect her boundaries.

"Jane's here," my receptionist calls.

"Send her back."

Hi.

"Hi."

So you might have some more questions for me?

"Hmm. Yeah, I do." I fumble for sticky notes on my desk.

"So how's it going on the meds and all?"

Well, the medications are very helpful, right on dosage and all. I'm more stable than ever. I'm doing well, and things are very consistent. Have been good for a while. I don't feel limited in any way except just take my meds and get a fair amount of sleep! And that's happening. It's been a climb.

Carolyn, try not to worry about me. You don't need to worry about the medication end of things. Dr. Jobson was so upset about what happened to me in Branson that he gave me his personal cell phone number. Jobson's smart, and so am I. Plus I read on everything like crazy. I think it's just a part of being able to communicate, especially with Dr. Jobson. He's excellent, and I think he trusts me. And he knows how capable I am. That man knows me. *Sometimes I ask a question, and he just stares at me, like I've knocked the ball right out of the park, really.*

"I know, I know, I know, Jane. But can't I be some sort of support in helping you go through this? Can't I be there to encourage, to remind you of hope, to be someone to reassure you in dark moments, someone to tell you when to slow down, and..."

Carolyn, stop. You're my therapist, *not my mother. I'll call you if I need to. I have you right here, right in my heart. You're precious. I'd like to see you again and again, but what you've given me is like a lifetime of love. It's great just knowing you're out there, that you care, that you are teachable. Somehow, I need to keep all of that deep inside me and, from the inside out, let my little light shine.*

"Little light?" I laugh. "Well, remember that, even if you can't *see* it, it's still there."

Thanks, Carolyn.

"You're done?"

Hmm. And you?

Jane smiles. I take a deep breath. I look away from her. My eyes well with tears, and I'm so torn. I breathe deeply, glad I have a book to write ahead of me. Maybe that will allow me to continue a relationship with her in some way or another.

Look, I told you I wanted to tell you my story. That's my story. I'm still working on how to explain to professionals and clients what they might do to help people like me, like the mentally ill. What can I say? Be yourself. Walk out your destiny.

Learn from difficulty. Pass it on. Stand up straight. Walk through the fire. Wear colored toe socks. Be proud. Change things up. Down-size...and every so often, like at a red light, think about what I've gone through and whatever I'm going to go up against in my who-knows future, which I think is gonna' be just fine! Ha! I'm going to handle it, Carolyn. Tell your clients to be tough, and teach them finesse and awareness. Carolyn, thank you so much, really.

"You're so welcome, Jane."

Jane rises and holds out her hand. Her grip is strong, and she looks good, not beaten up and tired from being with people who aren't kind. I didn't do much for her. Maybe I just didn't get in the way, but I also didn't fall asleep. That takes paying attention. Therapy requires finesse and talent and so many things that are often missing from our textbooks. Did that stuff get edited out, or have some important things not yet been published? Maybe people who are higher up overlook the obvious. That's a sin, an outright sin. I know that I can't be Jane's friend. I know I have to let her go, but one more question...perhaps the most important, for last.

"Jane, I've always wondered, you believe in God, but how does that work for you? I mean, how do you do it?" Jane looks me right in the eye and standing tall, she sits back down on the edge of her chair.

"How do you overcome, well, how have you...I don't know." I am saved by Jane who finishes my sentence for me.

How have I done it? I've answered it, my whole life was supposed to happen the way it has. Everything happens the way it's supposed to. There's a reason. We still have choices in most ways, though. I figured that God has a reason for making me the

165

way He did and putting me through it all. I just try to be obedient. And through God, I have peace and strength, and that's really all I need. We all have our battles to fight, our crosses to carry, our pain to grieve, our joy to weep, our efforts to find the light, our search for good. My life has simply been an effort to get it right. God helps, but it has really been hard. But never think that I don't have good, fun moments, because they're there. I've enjoyed much of my life even when I complain at times.

"I'm glad to hear that. So, Jane, why haven't you talked all about God to me?"

I have a bit. I've just tried to be practical and down-to-earth. He is in me and all around me. That's just how I see things.

And you know, it's not what we do in this life that matters, it's how we do it. Carolyn, you've done very well.

"You, too, Jane, you, too."

It's all about *kindness*, so simple.

Any Higher Power should be good, and any Higher Power would shower it all over everyone. Some people just don't absorb it. But there are as many concepts of higher power as there are people. I have a personal relationship with my God, and I don't criticize anyone else's ideas about their God. Simply put, God is what gets me through the day. And night. He is powerful, forgiving and loving. And that's what I try to be, through Him. When I carry Him in my heart or my back pocket, my life goes better. He has given me the strength to do what many people have considered impossible. See, it isn't I who is great. It is Him.

Whether I'm in a major crisis or just doing my thing in some wonderfully low-key way, it doesn't matter. Being with God has made my life Good. With God, even my worst pain is doable. He is awesome, Carolyn, not I. And I know I've hit a lowest low a couple of times, but somehow things are as they are. So even

166

though I've missed much in life and have been in what seems like
a constant rough go, sometimes afraid, He's there. My
relationship with Him, well, I couldn't or wouldn't ask for more.
I do get angry toward Him at times, especially when things are
hard and I'm wondering where the heck He is...but something
always draws me back to His grace. Carolyn, God makes what's
impossible possible.

"So then, how have you managed to talk with me,
write your story...without Him?"

Well, He's there. He's here. And Carolyn, like it or not, I
think that you are a higher power for me. I guess I'm saying that
God works through you. In my book, that's what He does.

I laugh at her pun. I smile into her eyes. Jane is so
vulnerable, so easily crushed and so human that it makes
me want to break down and just sit there, numb and in awe
of the greatness when one humbles oneself completely. It's
a paradox. It's as if she cares so much for others that she
somewhat loses herself, and she tells me that this is how
God intends her to be. Some people are destined to go the
two or even three extra miles, and Jane does it for anyone.
She's never been motivated to change that about her.

"So how and when did you find God?"

I guess maybe it's that, no matter where I looked, there
He was. I needed Him from the beginning. I don't know what
more to say. God is big, so big. He is just totally my best friend
who is there for me, especially when any human being couldn't or
wasn't. I've been broke, starving, homeless, jailed, hospitalized,
rejected, lost, at the end of my rope – all on several occasions, and
I've made out okay. I've done okay. If it's dumb luck, then that's
what God is at times.

What am I gonna' do if people see me for who I am? I've
been recognized as an athlete, singer, director...but this is about

mental illness, and that's very different. It's just going to be what already is, what's already been decided in God's mind. Carolyn, any book here is God's book, not mine. And you know, it might not sell. In that case, life goes on.

It's my job, my job, to serve Him, and He is just the most amazing friend and boss.

Once again, I, myself, am trying to comprehend how Jane's mind works. I'm trying to understand. Jane cares so much and has such passion. There's such a loyalty and freedom about her. Maybe our souls have met up. Her soul, I think, she wears on her very sleeves. No one can convince her that, in this troubled world, it should be any other way. I shake my being and come back to reality, envious of anyone she chooses for a connection, afraid for anyone who seriously crosses her. She has learned to take care of herself, which has been no easy battle.

Yes, Jane is a client. I'm a therapist. I know how important boundaries are. She never criticized me too much, and I came to trust her to tell me the truth, *her* truth. I also know how much I will miss her. I'll never forget her. Goodbyes are so important. Why must they hurt so much?

I'd trust her with *my* life. I'd turn my life over to her care completely. How is it that I feel I've always known her? How is it that she made *me* feel at home? It's so hard to figure things out. Jane smiles and says goodbye, and that's that.

I sit alone for several minutes, not quite ready to drive home. I turn off the light for the day and walk to my car. Lady is waiting for me at home. Walk? Total glee. I say goodnight to my parents on the phone, and then I watch the news, falling asleep with the TV on. After a while, I get up and go in the bathroom. I look in the mirror and realize that I probably won't see Jane again. And yet I feel a part of her within me, a part she had the courage to share with me. I run the shower for a wasteful but comforting hour and let the hot water cover me and soak into my 50-year-old bones. I think of one of the times she was in jail, pushing on the shower button, standing in an orange jumpsuit, just crazy about getting out...I laugh and sigh and have high hopes for her. She'll adjust. She'll set her mind to tolerating any light or any future struggle and be fine.

Okay, she'll just deal with things as best she can, whatever they may be. I'd say she almost has this whole life-long saga beat. I get out and towel dry, wondering if she'll ever give a talk as an expert and also tell her story. Maybe she will, and maybe she won't. I do think, though, that if she does, she'll have it easier getting on the right plane and wearing, maybe, a dress!

I need to get some sleep. Jane's story runs in and out of my mind as I toss and turn. Can she keep seeing clients, remain employed? Well, she hasn't missed a day of work in three years. And prior to her last medication/doctor upset, she worked 50-70 hours/week for eleven years. And prior to that, a medication/doctor upset, but 60-70 hours/week for five years of graduate school, a two-year post-doc... Can I even think to go through what she's lived? She loves to work...but seems to need to be her own boss. Or to have someone who gives her freedom and appreciation.

Maybe she and I are not all that different. She loves people but protects herself. She and I both have played a lot of things safe; we have little material wealth to show. She and I both care. We both know her story. In our sessions, we have visited a life of a woman that holds great meaning – someone ordinary who has lived her life in a way that is extraordinary. I ask, why is her life what it is, and mine what mine is?

No one ever really knows what past experiences will bring us to who we are today. That's okay. She shared her power and her vulnerability with me. She's a powerful mix of many good things. What's up with destiny?

And as for my anger and sadness over not seeing her again, well, that's how we come and go in each other's lives. The one thing that I'm sure of is something else she taught me:

Whoever we are,
    wherever we go,
        whatever we experience
           and whatever we feel,
our lives begin *now*. Our lives *always* begin now. And like Jane, every morning when I wake up, I check myself. I ask myself how I'm doing. And when I say 'fine' (yep, fine) and my feet hit the floor, I tell myself that I hope I have a good day. I wish that everyone could.

Each moment, I need precision and spontaneity so that I can move the right piece to the right place. I say: If only people wanted to do the right thing!

It's manipulation to force an outcome. If I do the right thing and then I do the next right thing, that is what love is about. When God tosses Jane the ball, she just tries to catch it. No, she goes all out to catch it. That's Jane. In her hard work, I haven't criticized her energy. I just hope she doesn't drink beer at all, and if so only *rarely*, especially being on medication, but somehow I trust her.

And I hope her friends and other people she meets are good to her, whatever that means, being there, staying out of the way, showing some support and

170

understanding...I hope that she has healthy connections. Relationships are what matter in life. I wish for her all the love possible. She told me one day that she doubts she'll ever remarry. Yet if she does, I hope it knocks her off her feet and gives her more freedom and joy than she can imagine.

She also told me that she fears someday being alone and unable to pay for medication or manage having a *home* of some sort. If she does end up homeless someday, I know she'll be okay. She'd end up in a shelter and have help and then an apartment, and if only they'd be sure not to leave out the antipsychotic med along with a mood stabilizer, she'd work...she'd shine joy into people's lives, I think so. I pause and then turn out my light.

***

I hope I can get some sleep, I whisper. *Don't worry yourself. Let everything go. Give it all up and rest tonight.*

The nightlight in the bathroom is bothering me. I get up and make my way across the room. I see myself vaguely in the light and through the steam still clinging to the mirror. I try drying the mirror with a nearby towel. It's not working all that well. My thoughts revert back to Jane. I think of what Jane said one session, about not being able to see her reflection in a mirror. She also told me one time that she was so crazy she thought someone else was living in her body, literally.

So who is it in the mirror? Who is looking back at me? I shake my head. I close my eyes. I think of that one psych unit, the many lights that formed the words in the middle of the night – in an office building: Thank you, Jane.

No, it said: Thank you, Carolyn. I touch the mirror with my hand. I press both palms upon the glass. I don't

171

think I'll ever forget that, at age 20? I won't forget being disordered. How could I? It's always there, a part of me. I think I will always have to monitor, always struggle, just maybe not as much. Hopefully, though, I can trust people whom I care about to help *me* moving forward in my destiny. Or maybe I can help *them*. It can go both ways. And you know what? It's really okay being Carolyn. I have no choice, and I am doing life as best I can. Maybe some people get that.

***

I have written a book about my therapist, myself. It's about, not two people, but one – one who cares and who has a lot to manage and who does so as graciously as possible. That's what a life can be.
And that's what it's been *for me.*

THE END

FACTS

There you have it – a glimpse of my life. I could have said so much more, but I will be writing a sequel and will have much to say at that point. The idea to write my life story came from my psychiatrist who, when I was 21 years old, suggested I write it someday. The format of this book came about, I suppose, because I have often felt like my own therapist. Or maybe I wanted or needed a therapist like "me" – someone who was patient and kind and who would work with me to build a life. Few people were willing (or should I say able) to help me accomplish what I set out to do each day. I "simply" wanted to overcome everything possible about my disorder. It has been a 24/7 job, every day of every week of every month for 33 years. At first, many people saw nothing productive coming from me, and no one really understood. I knew nothing to do but try to help myself. It has been a long and often painful, yet rewarding journey. What else could I do? What would you do? One thing I did do and still do is to *learn the facts*.

It helps to know the facts and the myths tied into a chemical mental illness. Myths are half-truths: information that sounds believable and might have been true at one time but is no longer so or never was true. We are now learning much new, fascinating and potentially helpful information about mental illness. Brain research is the most expansive area of new medical research today.

Here are some of the main facts to consider when it comes to what I call "chemical imbalances" or "brain disorders" such as schizophrenia, schizo-affective disorder, bipolar disorders and certain types of depression:

Fact 1: **"Chemical imbalances" are medical illnesses.**

This might be a stretch to accept, but it is important to break free of society's mindset. It might help you to see this when you consider the effectiveness of medication in addressing my delusions and hallucinations. Much of my disorder is medically treatable. I do not think that the medication numbs me (as might have been true in the past when the mentally ill were "treated" with earlier drugs) as much as it works to normalize my thinking and level out any extreme mood swings. I have other symptoms that I believe are medically treatable when treatment includes a diet that works for me. I consider certain foods to be helpful and others not. This is actually and simply my *opinion*.

Again my opinion: I do not think that there will ever be a diet as a cure, but the metabolism issues perplex me and seem complicated. It might be the case that I do so well due to medication, diet, exercise, sleep, taking care of myself physically, emotionally and spiritually. However, there is always going to be this lingering wonder in me about diet and mental illness, not as a replacement for medication but in conjunction with it.

Let me re-emphasize: The right medications for "chemical imbalances" typically work. They might not solve everything, but they are the driving force in a patient's journey to begin to heal. For those of you who do not consider "chemical imbalances" to be medical, consider that psychiatry is a medical profession that has changed radically as a result of the medications that are now the central aspects of most psychiatric treatment.

Fact 2: **Most violent people are not mentally ill, and most mentally ill people are not violent.**

The percentage of violent mentally ill people is not

much higher *or* is *not* higher than the percentage of violent people in the general population. You will find this statistic on many websites that discuss the stigma of mental illness. It's important to look at specific symptoms common to individuals who are mentally ill and exhibit violent behavior.

Mentally ill people who have "chemical imbalances" and who are violent typically suffer from command hallucinations such as voices telling them to harm someone. These few patients need to be on medication that can hopefully treat this symptom. If there is intent to harm another (or themselves) and they are unwilling to seek help and stay on their medication, they need to live in a setting where they will be protected from hurting others and themselves.

It is important for patients to know their own specific symptoms. For example, I have never had command hallucinations and have never been violent. I've never had thoughts of wanting to kill any other person. In knowing this about me, it might make it easier to interact with me. I hope so. And I hope that what you learn of others will help you know how you will interact with them, too.

There is another issue here. I said that some violent people are mentally ill. This violence might come about at any time, whether a person is psychotic, out of control or not. Why? Because some people are violent, and some violent people suffer from mental illness. Some violent people have diabetes, too.

Consider the flip side: In my own case and the cases of most, I am at risk of being a *victim* of violence when I'm disordered. I tend to run or hide when I'm disordered.

When I'm psychotic, I have always been able to stop when law enforcement told me to stop. Otherwise, they might have shot at me, who knows? I also could have run in front of a car. There are many predicaments that could be dangerous to me when I'm disordered.

It's a good thing that I know these things about myself. There aren't enough physicians who ask enough questions about specific psychotic behaviors. Sometimes I don't see how I have not been killed or seriously injured by someone out there who is ill intentioned; I lose the capacity to protect myself from society when I am disordered. Many people, even some professionals, don't seriously realize this. We, as a society, are often too busy being afraid of the mentally ill, especially when people are psychotic, when we need instead to protect them.

Law enforcement has helped me immensely. They contained me from running. They likely helped me from getting in with the wrong people. And they could tell I was sick. They make me nervous, but they've always been respectful and patient. I actually do better when they are the ones helping me and not friends or family.

There is a mental illness called Antisocial Personality Disorder (sociopath) in which the symptoms can include violence and lack of remorse as part of the diagnostics. This personality disorder is listed in the same diagnostic manual that houses schizophrenia, schizo-affective disorder, bipolar disorder and depression, which confuses the lay public and even professionals. It perpetuates the myth that the mentally ill, as a group of people, are violent or dangerous. It is my opinion that the illnesses I'm calling "chemical imbalances" should not even be in the same diagnostic manual as Antisocial Personality Disorder.

Usually, when a person who might be depressed and causes harm, there is often a personality disorder along with the depression that doesn't get discussed in the media. People with Antisocial Personality Disorder are people of their own right, but I think you can see the confusion.

Fact 3: "Bad parenting" does not cause "chemical imbalances".

Every parent is human and subject to making mistakes, but I'm not sure that there is any parental behavior that leads to these "chemical imbalances", not setting limits, chaos, drug usage, I don't know. Theory suggests that it is personality disorders, not "chemical imbalances", which result from certain parenting styles. At least, this was the theory when I was in graduate school. Studies of twins suggest there is more of a genetic component at work when it comes to "chemical imbalances". I have relatives who have suffered from mental illness, and a genetic explanation makes much sense to me.

I will say that it seems to me that Borderline Personality Disorder might be some type of "chemical imbalance" or at lease warrants medication at times, i.e., when they become psychotic. Also, a person with a "chemical imbalance" can also have a personality disorder, which needs to be considered in treatment. And there might even be a genetic component in these disorders, but as far as therapy is involved, the emphasis would be to help families learn to cope when their child or teenager who develops a "chemical imbalance" or any disorder a child or teenager might develop.

I do know that professionals need to be careful

giving children medication when the real problem is, actually, poor parenting and subsequent acting out. This is why assessment and a treatment team is so important when dealing with children and teenagers.

Any parent who focuses on, "What did I do wrong to cause my child to have this problem?" needs to redirect efforts to "What can I do to help my child cope with this illness, and what can my family do to help my child?" The presence of a "chemical imbalance" in a family adds stress, and the guidance needs to be solution-oriented, not blaming.

Fact 4: People with "chemical imbalances" are not necessarily emotionally weak.

Is a "chemical imbalance" an emotional weakness? Answering yes to this promotes the myth. I was a sensitive, compassionate and kind child. These personality characteristics followed me into adulthood. I do not consider them to be part of my disorder. Emotional instability, on the other hand, is a symptom of my brain disorder and is characterized by mood swings, which are highly respondent to medication. I can be high energy, and I also know the feeling of being depressed. But that is true of a lot of people. When medicated, I *am* high energy, but I typically love life and am very excited about it.

I put much time and effort into staying on track using willpower, self-talk, and so on. Also, I have a history that can be discouraging, with issues such as, *I'm tired of dealing with this. What do people know? Who is going to make life harder for me because of my illness? What does my future with my illness hold? Does anyone understand what I go through to be able to work each day? What more troubles am I going to create for my parents? How well could the strongest person do in my situation?*

Does this make me weak? I think it is a strength to think through issues and know oneself. No, I don't think I am weak at all. My experience has made me realize that a person with a brain disorder has to be tough, smart, resilient and responsible. For 22 years, I have been able to work hard and also manage my disorder. This requires a lot of strength.

I do think that I care too much about others at times; I have a lot of compassion and sensitivity toward others; and maybe that's a weakness or a fault. The Serenity Prayer helps me considerably in knowing what I can and cannot do when it comes to helping others. There are also times when, in feeling great empathy for a person, I have to tell myself that's enough, let it go. Anyone needs to have this skill.

In the story section of this book, anyone could rightfully say that I'm unstable, that I had costly upsets. However, look at what hung me up: developing my disorder at age 17 and not being diagnosed and treated until age 23; changing to another doctor who took me off the neuroleptic; another doctor who wanted me off it; developing tardive dyskinesia and poor medication management, etc. There were no instances of having trouble, i.e., being admitted to a pysch unit for any inability to cope with day to day or major stressors. What I'm saying is that I can be emotional, but I don't "fall apart" easily over emotional issues. Yet what if someone does? They deserve treatment for their problem, too.

When it comes to weakness or faults in clients, I try to help my clients identify their faults in a caring way,

179

because not knowing one's faults makes living with a ""chemical imbalance"" that much more difficult to manage.

Fact 5: Self-will or will power cannot overcome a "chemical imbalance" or brain disorder.

All the determination in the world cannot bring a person out of psychosis and into reality. If so, it's rare. I compare this issue to learning to drive a car. When I was first ill, I was all over the road. I learned to stay within the lines as best as possible, but psychosis and my other symptoms still prevented me from being a consistently good driver.

There were cues that I learned to take from people that helped me realize when I was "disconnected". This realization did not mean I *wasn't* disconnected. It just meant that I had developed an awareness that could, to a certain extent, help me stay safe and communicate with people about what I was experiencing. If my car breaks down, there is no amount of perfect driving that will fix it. Self-will is a great thing to have, don't get me wrong. However, it does not cure or treat a "chemical imbalance". I've always been strong-willed and tough on my mental illness, but when I'm disordered, I lose the capacity to be strong in the normal sense of the word. However, overall, it takes a lot of will power to try to overcome and live successfully with a "chemical imbalance".

Some people who have mild forms of a "chemical imbalance" might exert more control, but when someone is truly psychotic, I find it very difficult to use willpower to right oneself. I did reach a point of being able to talk when I was psychotic, and it was both helpful and confusing.

Fact 6: **There is a strong push these days to suggest that "chemical imbalances" are treatable (not curable).**

This is a loaded subject. With the many new psychotropic medications, the chance of a "chemical imbalance" being treatable is much greater than in the past. Yes, this is true. The medications are more effective, more specific and have fewer side effects. However, not all medical conditions are treatable, and the same holds true for "chemical imbalances".

I cannot find words to explain how difficult it has been for me to actually feel well and function well. My disorder may look treatable, but it has been all kinds of intervening and work that is ongoing and ever changing. It has been a full-time job, 24/7, for most of my life.

You might hear someone say, "Bipolar disorder is treatable," but I think we have to consider individual differences. The disorder needs to be broken down into symptoms that any given person might experience, and then medications and dosages that may alleviate those symptoms should be evaluated. Self-monitoring and knowing trouble spots are skills a person can learn in ongoing work with his or her doctor or a good therapist.

Here is an example: I once had a client who was diagnosed with schizo-affective disorder. He was on an antipsychotic medication, was somewhat in touch with reality, was capable of taking the bus to his counseling and could carry on a conversation. However, he heard voices that told him he was no good. I told him to keep trying, with the assistance of his psychiatrist, to find medications that might help with that. Meanwhile, I would ask him if he can ignore the voices, redirect his thinking and distract himself through activities, music, exercise, etc. I gave him feedback such as, "Hearing the voices is part of your disorder." I tried to help him take the power out of the putdown. He would ask me if I could hear them or knew that he is hearing voices. I tell him "No, thinking that I can hear them is part of your disorder." He told me that he likes to dance to music. But when he does that, his wife would tell him to go take his medication. I asked him "Do you think that your dancing is part of your disorder, or is it a hobby, a way to cope with the voices?" He said the latter. I told him to try explaining that to his wife and to have her come with him for his next appointment.

I do not hear voices telling me what to do. I have sometimes heard noises or muffled talking, especially as I'm trying to go to sleep. At age 23, I thought that others could hear my thoughts. My doctor successfully approached the problem from a medication standpoint. I have also found that, even when stable, I am very sensitive to any noises as I'm trying to fall asleep. Having a fan going helps tremendously with this.

There are also people whose symptoms of a disorder are more severe than other people's. We should not think less of people who have a "chemical imbalance" that does not respond well to a variety of medications. We should not assume that a symptom is psychological for the sole reason that it does not respond to medication. It is not the patient's "fault" if symptoms do not respond. It is important for the patient to work with the doctor to find a more effective medication. If that does not pan out, then consider that *new* medications not yet on the market might help in that patient's future.

***Fact 7:* Mentally ill people are not "bad" people.**

I run the risk of making a judgment call when I use the term "bad people." What I'm talking about has to do with *shame.* I will say this: Too many people who have "chemical imbalances" are ashamed and shouldn't be. Shame means feeling that one is a bad person. I used to feel embarrassed and ashamed of myself, especially when I was psychotic and realized what I had done. I was caught up and felt bad about myself, even though I couldn't control myself, which carries shame as well. We seem to think that thoughts, feelings and behaviors should be under our control at all times. When we lose that control, there is something wrong with us. When there is something wrong with us, then that is bad. We are bad. We feel ashamed.

Part of my shame is tied up with what I think other people think. I have made peace with my disorder to the extent that I know it is not my fault and can be explained medically. However, I know how a lot of people feel about mental illness, and sometimes I feel shame when I look at myself through their eyes. Let's face it: cancer survivors **receive awards** and are praised for their courage. People who have diabetes are **not** bad because of their diabetes. That does not seem to be the case with mental illness survivors. As a society, we need to **stop** shaming, laughing at and being afraid of mental illness. To do so is just plain cruel.

Fear fuels shame. We tend to distance ourselves from things we fear. We fight against things we fear. We fear mental illness, and we then tend to fear mentally ill people, even those who are harmless. This isolation can lead to people feeling unwanted and thus ashamed. There are times now when I still feel ashamed of myself, and I think it

183

has to do with stigma. I have become more loving toward myself, and I think that is what we all need to do for each other. There are certain behaviors that we should fear in one another, such as threats of harm and violence, but we cannot let our prejudice dictate whether or not we are willing to show support and care for those who need acceptance and understanding.

Bad things happen to good people. Everyone knows this, but we do not always know this in our hearts. I am a glaring example of how "a person as good as I am" can have a bad thing happen, such as my disorder. People like me are not supposed to have something that bad happen, especially not a mental illness. But genetics aside or maybe not, mental illness can happen to *anyone*.

I just wish people would jump in and be supportive so that the person with the disorder is not living the unnecessary nightmares – the ones brought about by ignorance and a reluctance to get involved and help. There is a hell on earth that we can dissolve if we carry love in our hearts. I cannot tell you how hard it has been for me to ask for help for fear of what people might think and decide about me.

Even as a therapist, often it is not easy to interact with someone who is psychotic. I sometimes feel inadequate in trying to converse with a psychotic person. They really need to have medication prior to beginning therapy. Instead of thinking in terms of bad and good, we need to think in terms of sick and well. We need to overcome our misgivings as a society and change our shame-based misconceptions. This requires deliberate action on everyone's part.

Fact 8: **Mentally ill people should not apologize for their behavior.**

I have worn myself out writing apology notes to people whenever I have done things when disordered. I had it all wrong for a good long while. After all, cardiac patients do not apologize for having heart attacks – even if they are overweight, eat the wrong foods and do not take care of themselves. Why then should I apologize for my symptoms? I should not, but it took a long time of chipping away at shame for me to come to that. I can be sorry for what has happened, and that is enough.

What about the many people who have put down patients like me – even my colleagues who say, "Oh shit, he's bipolar". I've heard my fill of callous comments. And what about careless professionals who have been wrong and who have caused me *harm* and *trauma* when they were supposed to help me? What about professionals letting me sit in jail for over a week when a simple phone call could get me to a hospital where I belonged?

Maybe I am not the one who should apologize. I should simply do my very best at protecting myself from my symptoms and try not to feel sorry, even though I so often have. There are patients who are supposed to take their medications but they are irresponsible and don't – maybe they should apologize. My point is that apologies are for being wrong, not for being sick.

Fact 9: **Mentally ill people should receive treatment, not jail.**

It would have been nice whenever my medications were changed and I ended up in jail if I had been taken straight to a psychiatric unit and put back on appropriate medication instead of spending a week in jail and in jail on more than one occasion – especially since I didn't break the

185

law. Being disordered is rough on me; it delays treatment. The longer I'm disordered, the harder it is and the longer it takes to get well again. It also creates memories that are hard to shake.

Putting me in a helpless position, both in jail and out and about, is dangerous. However, jail has its place. Law enforcement officers have helped me tremendously. I was not always taken to jail. There were times they took me straight to a hospital. They used *discernment*; they could tell. When I have been taken to jail, it does create a certain amount of safety. When I got the DUI, the jailers could see that I was sick as well as intoxicated, and they gave me a separate cell to keep me away from the other women. I was in no shape to be around others.

When it comes to crime, I still believe in doing the time, for the most part. I paid for my DUI just like anyone else, even though it was a case of self-medicating my disorder with two beers while on a road trip. It would have been nice if the court had taken the DUI off my record, but I got through it. Who knows – it might have helped to walk through the legal consequences in ways I can't see even now. In any event and for whatever reason, I broke the law. I was wrong, and I was guilty.

When it comes to violent crimes such as assault and murder, I do think we need to look at each case. I am all for making sure we keep everyone safe in our efforts to help the mentally ill. There are some potential problems, though. For example, some people are violent. Some violent people are mentally ill. In these cases, treating the mental illness does not necessarily address the violence.

Fact 10: **Once treated for a "chemical imbalance", you are**

not "good to go."

This is the case if your problem is chronic. Some people have one bout with depression, and that is it. However, if you have a problem that is chronic, there are numerous issues and you need to stay under the care of a physician and stay on your medication. For me, the struggle is ongoing and daily. I monitor myself constantly and have become an expert such that I am very effective in all I do.

Also, my medications and dosages have been changed at times. This is my reality, and I accept it. It is vital that you have a good connection with your doctor. There needs to be trust and partnership in discussing medications. As for psychotherapy, I do not believe it is required for everyone with a "chemical imbalance", although support and understanding from people are important. Taking care of oneself is a daily necessity, requiring focus and attention. I love feeling sane! Getting rest and being good to yourself is important. And what is wrong with that? Nothing at all, so just do it! If you have trouble and need to talk and get feedback, find a good therapist who has worked with the severely mentally ill. It can really help!

Fact 11: **Stress is a factor in almost any medical problem.**

Stress can even be positive, but like any good thing, balance is needed. Stressors can vary from person to person. Know what your stressors are. Knowing them can help you get and stay well.

For example, I find it stressful when I get up in the morning with only enough time to rush to work. My day is much less stressful when I give myself time to check out how I am feeling, go to work and create some mastery over my schedule and then deal with any difficult situation that might arise. I find that I do best when I go to bed at 8:00 p.m.. If I don't sleep well, I have more hours in which to get the rest I need. If I sleep well and am ready to get up at 4:00 a.m. or 5:00 a.m., then I have time to myself to write, read or watch TV.

I find it stress relieving to exercise, even if I do not want to at the onset. While working out, and almost always when I have finished, I feel stronger and more confident. I believe there is something about my metabolism that makes it difficult to do aerobic exercise, but I do enjoy walking, hiking, roller-blading and feeling fit. I do whatever I can. I connect with the outdoors or the person leading strength exercises on a video tape.

The most stressful situation for me is when I start to experience symptoms of my disorder. If I start losing sleep, it is hard not to panic. I cannot express how sad it is to feel my sanity crumbling. I do everything possible to get the sleep I need and stay on the diet I am on because then I can be "normal." If it means taking medication, then so be it. I am fortunate to have developed the self-awareness over the years that allows me to adjust medications, with the help of my psychiatrist, and remain exceedingly stable and on top of things in the workplace and at home as well.

I find it necessary to make sure that the people in my personal life are kind and caring. I set boundaries and refuse to enter a relationship with anyone who might "stress me out." I have some clients who are bipolar and who have lost jobs over not taking care of themselves in this area. I have tried telling clients who are determined to keep company with abusive people that they cannot effectively manage their disorders when in unhealthy relationships. For people with "chemical imbalances", there is no room to be sloppy in this area.

Fact 12: **Mentally ill persons can be employed.**

Anyone who has a brain disorder needs to figure out what he or she can and cannot do. I understand that most people who have my disorder, for example, are not employed. And I think that is too bad because employment can be very fulfilling. I think that a lot more people with brain disorders could be employed somewhere and somehow if employers were willing to help.

One of my biggest fears is not that I might be fired for screwing up. I do not make many mistakes, and never big ones. My biggest fear is that my employer might find out about my brain disorder and then find some reason, out of ignorance and lack of professionalism, to make life hell for me just to get rid of me. I try to stick with what I can do at any time in my life and go from there. Fortunately, my bosses have liked me and would likely be very understanding if they were to know my history. Those who have found out have been respectful and caring.

I have been able to remain employed in many jobs for long periods of time. Getting through college was rough, but once I was properly medicated, I did fairly well for a while. I worked my way through graduate school and carried a very heavy load for six years plus a post-doc position. When my medications were changed at that time, things became very difficult.

In Branson, I worked as a tech and moved up the ladder from there. I worked very hard at the treatment center for eleven years. Once again, having to change medications due to a serious side effect sidelined me. I started over as a tech while changing my counseling license and have done well for the three years since, having found a counseling position where I work full time and am not limited by my disorder. Taking jobs below my level of training has been part of *recovery* – mostly because those were the only jobs available but that also allowed me to get well and regain my full capacity. It pays to be smart in the world of employment. It has worked for me. I would encourage anyone with a "chemical imbalance" to find a workplace that is friendly and welcoming, even if other employees do not know about your illness. Find what you *can* do. If giving a job a chance is doable, do not let any myths stop you.

Fact 13: **Professionals may have "chemical imbalances"**.
      Yes, some of us do! There are physicians, therapists, attorneys, and many others who suffer from mental illness. Please understand how difficult it is for us to come forward. Unfortunately, many professionals do not seek the help available for fear of someone finding out that could lead to a job loss or any number of difficulties.
      I may be the exception to many rules in the nature and severity of my disorder, but I have always done an excellent job. When I am sick, I do not go to work. I do a darn good job of staying well, too. No one has ever had to counsel me out of a career or job. I have always known when to hold them and when to fold them, which was not often – even if this meant not having an adequate income or completely starting over at minimum wage, and even though I hold a PhD. Although I had to "start things over", I tend to believe people end up where they're supposed to

be. I also believe that everything happens for a reason. Maybe my reason is to help people understand mental illness, reduce the stigma, increase the awareness and point out stereotypes. And to have some fun amongst the difficulty of doing these demanding endeavors, when appropriate, while helping families who have endured great loss.

If you are a professional, understand that your decisions reflect and impact the rest of us. My jobs as a tech brought me joy, freedom, and a chance to focus on *me* in ways that are necessary and invigorating. House payments, cars, bills, kids – it is tough. See if friends and relatives will help. Downsize! Your kids might understand better than you think; they might just want their parents to be well! I tried not to worry what people might think as I moved a lot, never owned a home, took jobs below my education level, etc. It has been a lesson in self-love, as I battled shame for quite a while and still do at times. I also knew that I would likely never have children due to my illness, but this should *not* be a rule for everyone. I simply did not see myself as someone who could work *and* provide. Perhaps had I married early on and into wealth, I would have had kids and stayed home most of the time. I hate thinking about what kids go through when a parent is mentally ill, but love, understanding and family therapy can help.

When employed and carrying a caseload of clients, I *know* the importance of being stable and capable. It is because I am working with people who depend on me that I have very carefully moved into a job with this responsibility. I am aware of the need to be at my best, and my focus has always been to be on target for the sake of the people I serve. What has happened as a result is that I have

191

done very well, and people have been extremely pleased with my services.

It may seem like an excuse, but it is a *fact* that many of my providing physicians' sloppiness and even cruelty in managing my care have consistently resulted in a state of my mental disorder. Professionals who are supposed to help people like me should know that their negligence has cost me as a person and also as a professional. Dr. Jobson has trusted me and understands the concern I have for myself as well as my clients and peers.

I know a psychologist who is bipolar and who wrote an article where he said that, when he is experiencing added stress, he finds it necessary to increase his medication. It is his awareness and his partnership with an excellent psychiatrist that allows him to meet the demands of his own private practice while tending to his own health needs each day. I would think that his experience with his own disorder can be helpful in his work with clients. It is my wish that I do this, too.

Fact 14: **Prognoses are not set in stone.**

Better medications may allow previously untreatable illnesses to become treatable. We never really know when this might happen for a person, but it does happen. I also believe there are many actions besides medications that can improve a person's prognosis. I cover this in the Self-Help section of the book under *Activity.*

Be sure that you are telling your doctor as best you can what *symptoms* you are experiencing. Bring a caring family member or friend with you to your appointments if you feel information from them might help. Keep in mind that different medications may need to be tried. It was not until a doctor prescribed an antipsychotic for me that things started getting better.

I have more and more times when things feel normal. Diet as well as sleep patterns seemed related to these moments. I simply keep trying to do what seems to lead me toward better moments. When I was ill, I felt that I had nothing to lose. I did not let a diagnosis or prognosis stop me from trying to feel better through my own efforts.

Fact 15: Children can have "chemical imbalances".

There are children diagnosed with "chemical imbalances". There is, however, another issue of interest to me: In an adult diagnosed with a "chemical imbalance", were there signs of the disorder present in childhood? I am raising this issue as a result of what I experienced as a child.

My parents, who both had experience working with many infants and children, told me that my colic and insomnia were the worst they had ever experienced. The only thing that allowed me to sleep was if one of them drove me around in the car. I would finally go to sleep only to wake up and start crying again when they came to a stop and turned off the motor.

As a child, I remember having nightmares in which I was vomiting everywhere, only to wake up and step in the actual mess. I sometimes had trouble knowing if I had had a nightmare or if some event actually happened. I also remember feeling sick and shaky if I did not eat often enough. I passed out if I didn't eat, only to wake up later and feel fine. I did so well in school and sports that my pediatrician might have overlooked something possibly serious. Also, psychiatry was very different in the 60s as compared to now. It might have been better for me not to have been medicated as a child.

I do not know if my trouble sleeping and eating are part of my disorder today or if they simply co-exist with it. As a child, my pediatrician suggested I get involved in sports, which somehow seemed to tire me out and help. I don't know if there will ever be childhood markers that could identify adult-onset "chemical imbalances", but I wonder if such markers might move psychiatry closer to a cure for this particular set of disorders. Or at least allow us to catch it more quickly.

I started getting sick at age 16 or 17, and I don't really know if this is considered a childhood "chemical imbalance". I tend to think that I had onset symptoms that occurred much earlier, and we are better at picking up on such symptoms now better than ever before. We want to be sure of a diagnosis, however, as the label can follow a child everywhere into adolescence and adulthood.

Fact 16: **Brain disorders affect the people around us.**

Brain disorders may be a bit different from a less overt illness. I do know that my disorder has seriously affected people around me, especially when I am disordered. People who care about me seem to have a very tough time dealing with me when I'm disordered. My heart goes out to them. It has caused them stress even when I'm doing well. No one ever knows, for example, if a medication might need to be changed, and if I might therefore lose my income. One time, I had a professor who asked me, "What are you going to do if your medication stops working?" I told him the only thing I knew, which was to say, "I'll go from there."

Fact 17: **There is predictability in "chemical imbalances".**

I can say that this is true, but I am also 50 years old, so I have had many years of experience in learning this. The diagnosis of a brain disorder, by definition, tells you your general symptoms. However, different people with the same brain disorder can learn about their *specific* symptoms and patterns, which can then offer some degree of predictability. I go by certain rules of thumb that offer very real control – a sense of mastery. For example, insomnia, for whatever reason, is a red flag. It can lead to or be associated with psychosis. I have also found that, when I wake up and don't feel well mentally or physically, I usually feel better if I get up and get going. I know that I tend to do a better job than I think I do. I know that eating too much or eating the wrong food can ruin me for the day. A person with a brain disorder needs to look for patterns and predictability and work toward the goal of normalcy. Whatever you do, try to find good professionals to help you. Communicate with them as best you can so that they can help in your efforts to help yourself.

THE SIX A'S OF SELF-HELP

There are many suggestions I have when it comes to helping you deal with a mental illness and a "chemical imbalance" in particular. I am basing my suggestions on what seems to have helped me and what I have learned as a psychologist and therapist. I share what I know of myself as examples of what you might do when mental illness happens in you and your life. I do this with patients in mind. However, families and professionals might gain from my effort as well. These six A's of self-help are as follows: Awareness, Affirmation, Activity, Acknowledgment, Anonymity and Acceptance.

Awareness: I realized early on that I was "different," and I became particularly aware of this when I started becoming ill at age 16. People were calling me "weird," and I didn't know what to say or do. Sleep patterns, eating habits and my overall behavior felt out of control. I tried to understand myself. I continued to try to increase my self-awareness, awareness of others, awareness of my immediate environment and awareness of society – all leading to what I could change or do differently to make my life for me and others more manageable.

When I was 16 years old, I had a coach who was big on carbohydrates. Whereas a high carbohydrate diet was supposed to boost our energy, I found myself feeling sluggish, heavy and sleeping too much. My performance went downhill, and it was a shabby existence that turned worse. As I became aware of such symptoms, which I would later identify as depression, I also became aware that others were talking about me – some people were worried about me – and there was not a whole lot I or anyone else could do. I felt trapped.

In the throes of initial symptoms of mental illness, not much of anything helped. I understood, deep down, that something serious was going on. Yet I felt helpless. As time went on and as more symptoms arose, I could see that whatever I had walked into did not involve ever going back. I identified a whole host of glaring symptoms that tampered with any kind of life worth living.

By the time I was 21 years old, I was aware enough to know that I had a serious mental illness, one that would probably sideline me for life. My symptoms, which I primarily and reluctantly identified in my Abnormal Psychology class, included hallucinations, delusions, scattered thoughts, trouble expressing myself verbally, erratic sleep patterns, paranoia, mood swings, confusion, difficulty eating, not knowing what foods were right for me and anxiety.

I also knew that many people didn't and don't understand me. That's okay. Enough people did and do – enough people were there to help me and continue to do so. I made a decision to allow all experiences to teach me and help me live my life with my disorder. So in many ways, I have become an expert on being me, which isn't easy. I also have grown through the years as a person, and I'm not all that different from most people when my disorder is not active. People who know me well tell me that they would never know that I have this disorder if they were to see me for the first time today.

I have, at times, considered taking my own life. I didn't really want to do that. I just didn't see any relief, ever. I have learned that time alone can help. Things can change; things can happen around us that help our lives come together, even when we don't see it. It's imperative to allow for this, because there's no going back. In other words, we are not always aware of other workings in the bigger picture, workings I call faith and hope.

In having a brain disorder, I realize that my disorder is a *what*. I, myself, am a *who*. Even with symptoms involving my thoughts and moods, it is my *opinion* that it is still a medical disorder. And I still have a personality that is unique. We all do. I'm told the following things often: I'm honest, compassionate, forgiving, highly intelligent, insightful, patient, unwilling to give up, and tough on adversity. I'll go that extra mile for just about anyone. My friend Karen said something about me recently. She said that it's my kindness that stands out above anything else. I said, "How can you say that? I'm a type of genius." She said, "I know, but it's still your kindness that stands out." Another friend also said this exact thing. I was shocked, because I don't think of myself as all that kind – certainly not *that* kind.

I tend to be more aware of my character flaws than my attributes. I'm hard on myself, have done too much for people, often think the worst, feel like a second-class citizen, can be too sensitive, think people don't like me, am sometimes angry, hurt and scared when there's no point in being so. Some of my character flaws, I believe, stem from living in this society with my disorder.

My desire to help people, to be kind, and to strive for fairness are all attributes that still exist when my disorder is superimposed upon these traits. For example, when I'm disordered, I want to get all starving kids milk, pass out

198

fliers to help increase mental health conscientiousness, help inform people of an approaching tidal wave, make sure no one steps on my soul and set up an underground to help the mentally ill who are treated badly. My ideas and good intentions, which are part of who I am, are sound. It's just that my disorder imprints symptoms on my personality.

I have also become aware of other things about my disorder when left untreated: it is chronic; it leaves me vulnerable, a potential victim of crime and unable to care for myself; I shouldn't drive or try to go anywhere or do much of anything; I tend to want to self-medicate with beer; professionals look at me and minimize its nature. I have also become aware of 'red flags' – symptoms that suggest I need to take a look at my medication and dosages. These include fitful sleep, talking too much, pressured speech, flipping my days and nights, thinking too much, trouble focusing and remembering, confusion, hearing sounds and seeing things that aren't present, agitation. Over the years, I have become much more aware of initial symptoms and not letting things get out of hand.

It became vital for me to be able to explain myself to my psychiatrist in order to make *him* aware of what was going on with me. Outsiders, even trained professionals, do not always recognize when a patient starts getting into trouble until it's too late. Both a psychiatrist and therapist can be immensely instrumental in helping you learn about yourself and your disorder. This awareness can provide some sense of mastery and make life safer and disorders more treatable.

It is also important to become aware of your environment. Whenever I change locations, I know I need to find my way around. Any transition can be stressful for a number of reasons. I remember feeling overwhelmed at times with the simple task of punching in a new pin number at a pharmacy. I am also not sure how friendly people would be if I were to get confused and need help when out and about.

I've learned to take cues from others – sometimes people's reactions to me are the only clues to what's going on with me. For example, I might have trouble explaining an idea, and when someone else seems confused, I'm often determined to try harder and think things through. (For the longest time, when I was first ill, I practiced everything in my mind before saying it.) At other times, I think to myself, "I need to go home and get through these moments." I'm aware that, with many symptoms, time helps. I know how important it is, however, *not* to leave things to time when I feel certain ways – I might need to eat, to rest, to retreat to my room, take more of a medication, and hang on.

When getting used to new medication, whenever there's a change in medication, I pay as close attention as possible to any change in me. I need to be able to communicate what I experience to my treatment team. My anxiety is typically higher during these times, and so I expect that and tell myself to hang in there. I also try not to be *too aware* of details that aren't important.

Awareness is an essential part of monitoring how and what I'm doing, both from moment to moment and in general. It is a phenomenon that is always developing and is a necessary part of overcoming and living with a "chemical imbalance". And let's not forget, some things *are* confusing, hard to remember...and *anyone* can show certain symptoms when stressed or just having a bad day!

Affirmation: I have stated that my disorder is a *what*, not a *who*. An affirmation is a statement about *who I am*. It's meant to be positive and upbeat, something I can invent and learn to believe about myself. This is particularly important when it comes to "chemical imbalances" because there is prejudice toward the mentally ill and because the mentally ill often feel negative toward themselves. I tell myself daily, "I like me. I love me. I can make it." This felt awkward to me at first, but this kind of self-talk backed by a determination to be my best friend has helped me immensely.

My self-esteem took a beating when I first became ill, if only because my body was sidelined. I could not do what I had been doing, and I was afraid. It also seemed that others lost respect for me, ignored me and talked behind my back. I journaled frenziedly, telling myself to hang in there. *Writing* affirmations can be helpful. I often ask clients to draw and write affirmations on poster boards and put them on their bathroom mirrors. Sometimes I look at myself in my bathroom mirror and tell myself *I can make it*. It may seem uncomfortable or even stupid at first, but it can help.

As my illness progressed and I became aware of what I was up against, I began developing a sense of self-respect that is hard to explain. I could tell that my illness was not my fault or anyone else's, for that matter. My disorder became my challenge – what was I going to be faced with today, every morning, every night? What was it that I was asking of myself? I was asking for one simple thing – to do my best. And when I sometimes lost my footing and saw no hope, there was always someone in my life who *affirmed* my presence, my right to breathe, to stay in the fight.

Once I recognized the seriousness and severity of my disorder, my goals and values changed. Instead of determining that my disorder was forever disrupting my goals, I saw my disorder as my guide toward learning what I could and could not do. It was just a matter of locking in and trying some things until I met up with "defeat" and adjusted accordingly. Instead of grieving some loss such as sleep trouble in facing medical school, I said, "Okay, I can't do that. Learn and move on." I seem to constantly affirm the idea of finding my niche, having a place in life.

I sometimes chuckle about a social worker intern who admitted me to a psychiatric unit and asked me my religion. I told him that I was spiritual, and he said there was no box for that. I told him to *make a box* for spiritual. I do that every day – when I cannot find a place to exist, I make a place. When you get right down to it, my deepest and most important affirmation is: I like myself, I love myself, and I can make it. When I start feeling there's no light at the end of the tunnel, I remind myself as best I can that it's going to take *me* shining my light forward. Be your own light, shine your way forward to a better life.

Activity: At times, my fears have immobilized me. There have been times when I thought no thoughts, felt no feelings, and remained motionless. I know of days when my racing, broken mind overwhelmed me to my wit's end. I remember waking up and not caring if my bed burned to the ground – with me in it.

Momentum helps, it seems. If I can get going, I might stay going. I let my life pass me by for only a moment. I have to face my day, even if that only means clutching a mattress and rolling over every few moments.

My connections to the moving world can be sparse, especially when I've crashed and burned. Being disordered is exhausting.

I *try* to get up and go to group or work, depending where I am. I *try* to talk. Words come out in the wrong order. *I keep trying*. I read self-help books. I push myself spiritually. I commit to a partnership with my psychiatrist and explain my symptoms as best I can. I show up for therapy. I don't allow others to define me. I keep track of food. I learn what to eat and when to eat and how much to eat and what food helps with what symptoms. I exercise. When I feel stuck, I try my best to change things up! Do something different, try to find what works when! I mess with my chemistry with food, exercise and sleep schedules, in often desperate efforts to get out of the mess my disorder has me in. I talk about these things with my psychiatrist. And I ride that bronco 'til it throws me. When it does, I dust myself off and get back on. More than anything, I tell myself that I belong on this earth, and I need to see myself through.

Staying active is one thing, but not everyone who is mentally ill is capable of employment. Staying symptom-free is not easy. There may be some kind of work, however, that you *can* do – flexible volunteer work, for example. It's also possible that a person with a "chemical imbalance" can work around illness with an employer. Taking college or on-line classes are possibilities as well. Don't let society convince you that there's absolutely nothing you can do. This world is meant for all of us. Lest we forget, people with chemical imbalances can have other illnesses as well. I know of a woman who has both schizophrenia and breast cancer.

I let people help me. That is my biggest burden of all, being a burden to others. But it's a burden worth carrying. Let people help *you*.

Acknowledgment: Not *every* moment is painful. I grow to appreciate the better moments and try to learn from *all* moments. Some moments are highly embarrassing while other moments are shame-filled, anger-filled or seemingly impossible. I have not forgotten that many moments are *good* when compared to the tough times. Some moments are downright dangerous and life threatening, and it's not as if I *choose* to be in harm's way. Many desired outcomes seem unattainable and are just that, and so I move on – around, under, over, any which way. My disorder has severely limited me, but I've simply tried pushing limits in an intelligent fashion.

I hung in there and somehow have made it to "today," maybe in part because I did see the good moments. Maybe it was because I wanted and needed to *learn* about me, my predicament and my disorder. I have tried hard to be the best person I can be.

When it comes down to it, we are each responsible for managing our own health, that is, if we are able. Some people with mental illness need someone to hand them their medications, keep a close eye on them, go to the doctor with them, and so forth. For me, I manage my health and my illness, but I have *help*. And it's up to me to utilize that help. I rely on a psychiatrist, friends and family. At one time when a psychiatrist was many miles away, I relied on an internist to prescribe my medication. (I wouldn't recommend an internist for helping you change medications.) At times, I've seen a therapist, and I recommend it whenever you can afford it. It's great to have someone to talk with freely.

In managing my health, I realized that I needed to *admit* that I have a problem. I don't like the harsh reality of having schizo-affective disorder, and I did not want to hear those words from my psychiatrist when I was originally diagnosed. Deep down, I knew that I had some form of schizophrenia, but it helped me, for a while, to deny it. I knew that I had a serious disorder, and I knew enough to take my medication. I knew that my prognosis was not great. And so, I called it a metabolic disorder or an atypical bipolar disorder, names that sounded more in line with something I could conceivably conquer.

Why me, I asked early on. I don't seem to fit the stereotype, whatever that is. I am intelligent, talented, and caring; I certainly don't deserve it. Why me? Because I can handle it? Because I wear my illness well? Because it makes me a better person, a stronger person? Because I have something to offer people in having it? I don't know. Maybe the better question is, "Why not me?" Why can't a kind, loving and smart therapist have schizo-affective disorder? Apparently, she can. She has worked as such for 22 years, brilliantly and with great compassion.

One advantage I have over a lot of people is that I've been evaluated and know my mental health. I've made it back from insanity several times, and I don't have the worry of many people and therapists, such as *Oh, how embarrassing to go crazy. Will I be doomed? How will I manage?* I've overcome many fears others have yet to reckon with. I've been embarrassed; I've been doomed; I've not managed. Yet here I am! I also have had to work so hard to gain every ounce of mental health possible that I'm mentally healthier than many people. Now that's a paradox. Put in more understandable terms, I've taken such good care of myself that I rarely get sick in any way, and I'm typically in a better mood than most people despite my troubles.

Of course, I struggle. My worries just might not be exactly the same as yours. They needn't be. We don't have to be the same to get along. However, we can all strive toward better mental health practices, and this involves getting educated for your own sake but also for your neighbor's. I grew up with the idea that you need to keep your problems at home and not tell your neighbor. The only trouble with that was that I would get on the phone or take off running out the door. Oops!

Surely there is meaning and purpose in life – we need meaning and purpose, and one of the joys of life is finding your purpose, *creating your* purpose. Since I've lived a life of driving backward and looking in the rear view mirror, I don't know my purpose. But I do think that everyone's life has *some meaning*, and I'm not convinced we need to see it at all times for it to be present. One of my purpose's has been to be a good family member and a good psychotherapist. Perhaps there are more.

Anonymity: Some people with "chemical imbalances" choose to tell others about their disorder. Why? Perhaps they think nothing of it and talk about their health with anyone. I suggest that patients put some thought into *whom* they tell, *what* they tell, *how* they tell and *why* they tell. It seems to me that it would be difficult to keep information away from family, unless there's no contact with family. In my case, my parents know. Some close family friends know. My friend, Karen, in Branson knows as do the people with whom I worked in Branson. Anyone who has known me in a medication or doctor change knows. My psychiatrist knows. My internist knows. Some people at Vanderbilt know.

The question is what do they know? They each know only bits and pieces, that's all. Telling everyone is a personal decision and should be thought through. I inform people on a *need to know* basis or for a really good reason.

Sometimes it helps to talk about your disorder and symptoms. Call it *venting*. Call it *accessing feedback* from others. Call it *staying on track*. Call it *learning about oneself*. Professionals, family and friends can help with this. I have read books written for families and friends that seem to suggest how to deal with symptoms rather than how to deal with a patient with symptoms. I like to think that patients, for the most part, can guide others in helping to understand their disorders. In this light, there are as many people as there are disorders because the patients who are in the driver's seat can teach and share what may be helpful for themselves and others.

It may also be up to the patient to provide *reassurance* for others. I can tell people close to me, for example, that I'm having some trouble sleeping or I am not feeling well today. My point is that information should be shared that minimizes stress on the patient and others. For others, once some level of reassurance is provided, it is up to them to trust, let go and see how things go. I might also say to my psychiatrist, on a more detailed level, that I'm seeing things in my peripheral vision, for example.

When I feel particularly bothered over not knowing who knows what, I sometimes tell myself that everyone knows everything, and so what? This approach takes the bite out of paranoia. I also ask myself, what's the worst thing that can happen in people knowing? They'll run me out of town? Who knows – there may be a showering of praise over my lifelong efforts. I don't really know.

In Branson, when people found out my medication had been changed, they showed understanding and acceptance. There were people who still hired me; there were clients who still sought my services. So it's hard to know what people and other professionals might say and do. I hope I'm spared the shame and humiliation I've endured in the past. I do hope that my story, and my risk of presenting myself, might be of benefit to others. I'll walk through fire to help a person I don't even know! And it's not that I'm a great person; it's that I know the damage mental illness can do and does. And I know I'm in a position to do some possible good. I wrote my story for myself. I got it published for others.

Acceptance: These past three years have been a real fight for me in adjusting to medications, mopping up the mess and holding down a job. Can you believe it – the mess that happened over a little change of medications?! Getting used to the new regimen has felt like World War II to me, but I feel that overall I'm winning. Unfortunately, I didn't have immediate access to my doctor, and that was costly.

So how have I managed? It hasn't exactly been a crap shoot, but especially early on, things *were* hit or miss. I had to focus on any moment of clarity and normalcy, and build on that. I always worked toward getting my disorder to be *treatable*. That is my daily goal today and always has been. At age 50, I'm saying, "Oh, wow, God is amazing." Even in my toughest and seemingly most hopeless moments, I felt His miraculous presence, no matter the situation, no matter the outcome. I've worked hard on myself, praying for strength and guidance every day.

I've figured out the mind over matter issue – what you should do when your mind goes haywire. I know what I did when I was crazy and exhausted. When I was first ill and had moved back in with my parents (and when everyone else was going to college), I asked for a guitar. My mom said, "Well, only if you'll play it." I knew I would, because it felt as if that's all I'd have. I sat on my bed and played for hours. I sang with some inner voice that I could hear through the music. I think it was an inner voice that I could identify even when I was disordered. Maybe it was another part of my brain that I kept alive.

I practiced the guitar every weary day, and it brought an ounce of sunshine into my world. Not every fiber of our being is crazy when we're mentally ill. Part of our spirit remains untouched and free. Harnessing that energy sets us free and apart from feeling trapped. My guitar knew no limits, and I didn't try to be the best in the world at anything. I just tried to *belong* in the world. I hope that you, too, can learn of your own belonging and find some joy in this world.

AUTHOR'S NOTE AND ACKNOWLEDGEMENTS

I don't have a lot of people to thank unless I decide to simply thank everyone. I do know that people in my life have more or less come and gone. It seems that people in my life who have helped me in some way or another have been there at the right time. Even some of the rudest, meanest people have actually helped me. However, I'll stick with those people who have loved me when it comes to thanking.

***

I want to thank every teacher and coach who cared. They never tired of encouraging me, in both my best and worst moments.

***

Every mentally ill patient, tucked away in our shame-filled state hospitals and jails from Day One, I thank. You are truly my life and my love, and we should yearn for your forgiveness.

***

All of my relatives, especially the ones who lived the most of their years in hospitals or who seemed very depressed or unable to live alone, I thank. You are truly my heroes, and I am proud to be your family.

***

I want to express my gratitude for my most enduring pets: Muffin, Brecken, Bo and Lady. Their capacity for love has been consistently unconditional and perfect. They were and are there for me every step of the way.

***

I thank E. Fuller Torrey, author of Surviving Schizophrenia, for all he has done in the field, which is huge, and for reading my manuscript and seeing its worth.

***

I want to thank my sister Connie for demonstrating that a sibling of a person who is mentally ill can soar and have the best life possible. I want to thank her for showing me that the sky is the limit and that relationships can last forever. I also thank her caring husband Adam Lehman and her two wondrous kids Sam and Grace .

***

Karen Kramer, a substance abuse counselor, continues to be my very best friend. We have shared ins and outs, ups and downs, always there for each other if even on the phone and across the miles. The number of people she has helped, while remaining so humble, is astronomical. She has been an awesome role model. My admiration for her abounds. Her steadiness has often guided me. Her spirituality has helped her overcome much and has taught me. She is a true friend for life. Thank you, Karen, for *everything*.

***

In 2009, when I asked Cathy A. Kodra, A freelance editor, writer, and member of the Board of the Knoxville Writer's Guild, to edit my book, I had no idea that I was going to meet one of the most talented, diverse women in the writing field. She worked with me on my first book writing project and encouraged me to meet up with a publisher. Cathy's editing skills are excellent and she worked patiently with me. She has strong and insightful editing skills and offered much valuable and helpful feedback. Yet what also makes her special is her patience, integrity and dedication to helping others. Cathy has encouraged me every step of the way and I trust her implicitly. I am grateful and honored to know her. If I were to write a sequel, there is no doubt I would work with her again to be my editor. Thank you, Cathy, for *everything*.

***

My psychiatrist, Dr Kenneth O. Jobson, is brilliant, kind and supportive. He never spared me the truth when I asked him question after question and made suggestions for myself. He never tried to limit me in my professional endeavors and never discouraged me, ever, from trying. He encouraged me to overcome the instability with my efforts – whatever it is that I do – alongside medications. He has told me over and over that I'm brilliant, especially when I felt like an idiot. He has applauded me for the wisdom and expertise that I've developed. I have known him for 31 years, and I consider him, not just my doctor, but a true friend. I'm proud of what he's done to help me, what I've done to help myself and what he and I have done together.

***

George Tinkham, a substance abuse counselor, has quite a sense of humor, has been the kindest friend and amazingly dedicated staff person. He's someone I would trust with my life. It's been a joy working with him and knowing him. Thanks for the good times, for being there and for never judging me.

***

Thanks to Anna Mason, as I had the joy and pleasure of watching her grow and develop a wisdom and confidence that has me in awe. You have been a role model and have helped so many, and I miss your trust and kindness. Sometimes I think you can't possibly be any better, and yet you keep growing and being a miracle in people's lives.

***

If I'm to have a cause, I guess I'd be thrilled if people could see my faults as well as my strengths and be okay with them. I wish we would treat the mentally ill with some elevated kindness and understanding through what's in my book. If my book helps with that, I'd be standing in the back row unnoticed – mixed in with everyone but clapping the loudest.

***

A special thank you to Marvin Ross of Bridgeross Communications for believing in me, being extremely patient and especially for having his heart in the right place. Thank you, Marvin, for your professionalism, your undying enthusiasm, your passion and your dedication in "the cause". You are a true believer.

***

And honestly, I'm clapping for Jesus Christ who has been *my* Strength, *my* Brother and Father, *my* Role Model and *my* Light, One that has kept me going and One who would be saddened if I were to ever forget His importance *to me* and *my* cause, as I know it. I thank Him for making such a difference in my humble, imperfect life where I can only be given credit for trying to be a good person.

TO MY COLLEAGUES

I know of several highly educated, accomplished professionals who have contributed greatly and who also suffer from some type of mental disorder: three psychologists, an attorney, a nurse and three physicians. One of them has bipolar disorder, two of them have depression, two have schizophrenia, two have schizo-affective disorder and one has borderline personality disorder.

We're living in a time when quite a few professionals are coming forward and telling people about their mental illnesses. For example, on National TV a few months ago, a neurosurgeon lost his marriage and father in a couple of months time, went into a deep depression and had to quit work. He got help and is back doing neurosurgery. Here are other examples: I know of a physician who hears voices. I also know of a nurse who works all day but has suicidal thoughts each evening.

My guess is that most people would not want to be under the care of these health professionals. If I'm wrong, then we can all go home. In my opinion, these professionals have wonderful minds and brave hearts. I don't think they're coming forward completely for their own well-being. The risks are there. I believe that these professionals put quite a bit of thought into their decisions and how coming forward might play out. I also believe that they came forward for the right reasons: Because they care. Or because they refuse to make the stigma a bigger deal than they believe it should be.

If someone asked me if I would want to be treated by

any of these professionals, I would say that I want the best. If they happen to have a mental illness, then so be it.

So then maybe the next question is: Can a professional *really* have the judgement and other needed skills to actually do the job of these professionals I mentioned? My answer is: Some can, and some can't. It would depend on the person, the skills needed, the symptoms, the stability and the employer. Hearing voices has not prevented this physician from doing her job. For some, it might. I'm challenging you not to make assumptions.

There are some truly amazing professionals who can endure their difficulties and contribute brilliantly. We should applaud these people. Actually, we should applaud anyone for trying. We should encourage everyone to try. And if the job cannot be done, I would want that professional to try for something else. This decision concerning job capacity should be made under the care and opinion of that professional's treatment team.

It is our ethical responsibility to avoid the "we and they" mentality, do away with outcome expectations based on diagnostics and exercise some open-mindedness. It isn't easy to be mentally ill, and it isn't easy not to be mentally ill. Better said, for many, *life* is not easy.

Hear what I'm saying: a person can have the same disorder as someone else, but due to individual differences, each person might aspire to vastly different levels of competence – even in the same job. If we do not consider individual differences, we are sending a wrecking ball through the very awareness and understanding we so desperately need to develop.

I don't know for certain why each professional

comes forward. Some have said that it gives clients hope. I learned in graduate school, for the most part, that we aren't supposed to tell our clients a whole lot about ourselves. Well, I'll tell you when that went out the window for me and why.

During these past few years, I was finding myself very restless, dissatisfied and tired of a certain mentality that I have faced every day for 25 years. It has to do with stereotype. In meeting me when medicated, no one would ever think I had a mood disorder and certainly not a thought disorder. Yet I kept my mouth shut and said nothing when a peer would tell me "You don't want that client; he has schizophrenia". And in the same breath, I was being told by that peer that he wished I were his therapist. So I sat there, hearing such things, for years. Up to a point, it didn't bother me. We're all human.

Then it did start bothering me in a huge way. I was realizing that many professionals were not getting the help they needed, because someone might find out and think of them as less competent, thus affecting their jobs and incomes. Others were simply in serious denial.

I wanted to do something about this. I wanted to help. So one solution for me was to write that book I've had in the back of my mind for 30 years. I wanted to address the fear, and one way of doing that was to say, "Hey, you want to see mental illness, well, let me tell you..."

See, I have been mentally ill since age 16, and so the issues of my colleagues' predicaments didn't exactly apply. Nonetheless, as I was in the process of becoming a doctor, I realized that there is a pressure for the professional to be well while the client is sick. So how then could I become a doctor? It happened, because I did the work. People like me don't have schizo-affective disorder...why? Because it's stereotyped that way. Because overcoming the symptoms is rough.

I think that maybe, like me, a lot of professionals have had enough of the hypocrisy and putdowns. Here's the catch: These disorders we have can often be treated. Even if not, some people can adapt to the symptoms and function quite well. And more could, if we would teach them, teach them not to be so afraid.

My book is about respect, and my book is my truth, stories of things that have happened to me, things that I have done. I tell my story, because seemingly selfishly, I want people to change. As this book project progressed, however, I'm learning that it has been anything but selfish. I lived freely and quietly for years, and I was going to give that up? Why?

I said to myself, "I wish I knew then, in high school and college, what I know now. And I sure would like to make things easier for my colleagues, the ones who need help." And it's that simple. There are teens and young adults and professionals, this moment, who are depressed, developing schizophrenia, cutting on themselves...and what can I do to help them bypass much of what I went through? I learned a whole lot from ages 16 to 50, and it is there for you if it might help.

I want people to have every chance for freedom without ignoring the true limits their disorders place on them. Times are changing, but throughout my life, professionals often set limits on me based on diagnostics. It still goes on. I know the pains and difficulties of mental illness. And stigma is much of it. One way to fight stigma is to explain. I felt compelled for a couple of hundred pages.

I have served in the mental health field for 22 years, and some voice from within me said, "Enough. Enough." I was willing to risk who-knows-what for the sake of trying something different. At one point, I thought things couldn't possibly be worse concerning the secrecy. I knew that coming forward in my book could really be tough, but the silence was worse. It had grown to be as such over the years.

People are looking for answers, hope, encouragement, support and strength. I hope that my book might help someone say, "She did it, so can I". I'm not talking about having a PhD or being a top athlete. I'm talking about being yourself, following your dreams and understanding that some people are going to assign limits to you based on your disorder. I suggest that you resist this. I suggest you focus on being as symptom-free as possible.

If someone, even a professional, tells you that you can't accomplish something because you have such and such disorder, you ask that professional to explain and then head toward decision-making with a competent professional. For example, there was a psychiatrist who, because I was in graduate school, told me I could not possibly have schizo-affective disorder. In this case, I was stereotyped and not considered an individual.

I bought into into his know-how, and it was costly. Early on and especially after these kinds of experiences , I vowed to learn everything I could about my disorder and myself. In my learning process, I started taking charge and argued with professionals who were hurting me. It's a rough go, so be prepared. I, for one, am glad I've hung in there. As an adolescent or professional, seek out good help, especially if your disorder is particularly difficult.

The truth of the matter is that, with the new drugs, the movement to reduce the stigma, the increased knowledge and understanding, the craving for awareness, and the people stepping out, there will be more and more people who will hopefully find better help, will get better help and will live more productive lives. Most importantly, we all might be able to do so without such worry about what people might think, say and do.

There will be more people who will not go through all of what I went through. That brings me joy and hope that they can find their own happiness. We are moving in the right direction, but we need to do more, be more proactive. I am proud to be a part of this development – mental illness becoming easier due to eradication of the stigma. And if more people join in the fight, mentally ill or not (as it affects us all), then we all reap the benefits of being part of the solution. That cannot help but lead us to leave behind the kind of fear that holds us back.

AFTERWORD – Dr. Kenneth O Jobson

Carolyn Dobbins, PhD lives a life of vitality and value despite a Schizo-Affective Disorder that has led her into multiple thought and mood symptoms and a state of psychosis when not properly treated.

With determination to mange multiple symptoms, she came to understand the necessity of a multi-faceted approach toward wellness, that is, addressing her illness from several standpoints.

With dedication and a pledge to true partnership in her treatment, she has become a lifelong learner.

Proper medication adherence has been key to her progress. Psychotherapy has been substantial and focused. Manyfold monitoring was utilized, and she participated with excellent communication and contingency planning.

She relied upon medical lifestyle management and preventive care, including diet and exercise. She maintains a psychological attitude of mindfulness, appreciativeness, hope and love. Like a general, she deploys big heartedness and tough mindedness amid the rest. She is successful in learning how to live her life.

This book gives a model of resilience and success in dealing with a troubling and potentially lifelong disabling psychiatric illness - a model that conveys a strategy of action and attitude. It can serve patients and their families toward tackling demanding expectations and experiences with severe psychiatric illness. It informs and gives one hope.

Kenneth O. Jobson, M.D.
Psychiatry and Psychopharmacology

BIOGRAPHY

Carolyn received her BS from University of Utah and her PhD from Vanderbilt University in 1990. While at Vanderbilt, Carolyn received an NIMH scholarship and two two-year Clinical Fellowships along with four research assistantships and a research associateship.

Carolyn has served in the mental health field for 22 years.

She helped develop a co-occurring treatment center and co-directed it for nine of the eleven years she worked there.

She has primarily been in private practice, working mainly with teenagers, clients with substance abuse issues and clients who have major mental illnesses.

In her teens, Carolyn was a top, nationally ranked Alpine skier until age 16-17 when she began developing a major mental illness. At age 23, she was diagnosed with a chronic and severe Schizo-Affective Disorder.

Carolyn has written and has had published *What A Life Can Be* in hopes it might be helpful to any reader. In coming forward with her book, she has become available to speak about major mental illnesses, her knowledge and her experiences.

Carolyn currently lives in Knoxville, Tennessee, has a private practice and is a member of the American Mental Health Counselors Association. She is licensed in Tennessee and Missouri.

COMMENTS ON THE BOOK

Carolyn Dobbins' account of her own Schizo-Affective Disorder is an inspiration for all who have ever experienced psychosis. Despite her symptoms, she is able to move her life forward and now practices as a psychotherapist helping others similarly affected. It is very well written and highly recommended.
Dr. E Fuller Torrey, Author of Surviving Schizophrenia

Dr. Dobbins gives us an honest, heart-wrenching, and sometimes humorous look deep into the life of a woman with a severe mental illness. Beyond its intriguing value as a "good read," *What a Life Can Be* is a strong step toward more understanding, support, acceptance, and hope for those who struggle with mental disorders. In my interactions with Carolyn Dobbins, I often forget that she, indeed, suffers from a mental illness. A respected psychotherapist with years of professional and personal experience in her discipline, Dr. Dobbins is a skillful writer who offers the best of the best: both sides of the fence, and what we *all* can do to make things better.
Cathy A. Kodra, Freelance editor and writer, Knoxville, TN

As one of Dr. Dobbins' graduate student professors, I can attest both to the uncommon talent and the painful life of this exceptional therapist, patient, and author. Her story is powerful and revealing, and provides a unique insight into chronic mental disease. She has has the rare ability to understand chronic mental illness through both a developing insight into her own disorder and the expertise of a doctoral level psychologist. Her book is a probing, honest, liberating story.

Tom Burish, Provost and Professor Of Psychology, Notre Dame University

Carolyn's story is inspirational and encouraging to those who have major mental illnesses and those who do not. She tells of her life and experiences in a way that reflects a warm and kind personality. She was my supervisor and has been my friend for almost ten years. Her writing is real and down to earth, and she has much insight and much to say about mental illness and people in general. She has been a true friend, which is rare, whose kindness and intellect shine through. I am blessed to know her and would trust her with my life.

Karen Kramer, Master's Level Substance Abuse Counselor, Former Associate Director, Branson, MO

I made the acquaintance of Carolyn Dobbins in 1998. She has been my co-worker, supervisor, mentor and friend. I quickly became aware of her devotion to her profession and a strong dedication to clients' well-being. She has exhibited an intense desire to do what is right, not only when it comes to her colleagues but to anyone she comes in contact with. The reader will benefit as greatly from her knowledge and deep insight as all of us who have worked alongside her at one time or another. She shows us that it's time to dispel the stigma and fear of mental illness replacing them with tolerance and understanding.

George Tinkham, Substance Abuse Counselor

Long before I was given the opportunity to work with this

dynamic lady, she saw something in me that I could not yet see in myself. As an addict in early recovery I found her spirit and energy to be inviting...something I wanted back into my life. She encouraged me every step of the way and when the time came, she challenged me to be something more under her supervision. Even though our time together ended years ago, I continue to be inspired by Carolyn and the respect she has for life.

Anna Mason, CADC, Substance Abuse Counselor

SIMILAR TITLES FROM BRIDGEROSS

Schizophrenia Medicine's Mystery Society's Shame by Marvin Ross - recommended by the World Fellowship for Schizophrenia and Allied Disorders. "a powerful resource for anyone looking for answers and insight into the world of mental illness." Schizophrenia Digest Magazine, Fall 2008

After Her Brain Broke: Helping My Daughter Recover Her Sanity, by Susan Inman. A poignant memoir describing the family's nine year journey to help her younger daughter recover from a catastrophic schizoaffective disorder and recommended by NAMI.

My Schizophrenic Life: The Road to Recovery From Mental Illness by Sandra Yuen MacKay. "Inspirational and fosters some hope for recovery", Canadian Journal of Occupational Therapy; "remarkably compelling", Library Journal and recommended by NAMI

The Brush, The Pen and Recovery, A 33 minute documentary film on an art program for people with schizophrenia. "I loved this film. Without shying away from the realities of having a serious and persistent mental illness, three courageous people talk of their struggles, their dreams and their hope. Educational, accurate, human, and compelling." Dr Peter Cook, Department of Psychiatry & Neurobehavioral Sciences, McMaster University

CPSIA information can be obtained
at www.ICGtesting.com
Printed in the USA
BVHW03s1736220718
522322BV00001B/26/P

9 780986 652226